Praise for the *Voices of* Book Series

"Pure inspiration."

Shape Magazine

"...provides answers to practically anyone wondering 'What now?' ...this worthy collection succeeds very well."

Publishers Weekly

"Hearing others' stories is the most substantial aspect of any support group... It's the universality of the emotions that links these essays and puts the human face on what can be a very scary disease. For all patient health collections."

Library Journal

Other Books by The Healing Project

Voices of Alcoholism
Voices of Alzheimer's
Voices of Autism
Voices of Breast Cancer
Voices of Lung Cancer

Voices of Caregiving

The Healing Companion: Stories for Courage, Comfort and Strength

Edited by

The Healing Project

www.thehealingproject.org

"Voices Of" Series Book No. 6

LaChancepublishing

LACHANCE PUBLISHING • NEW YORK

www.lachancepublishing.com

Copyright © 2009 by LaChance Publishing LLC

ISBN 978-1-934184-06-6

Managing Editor
Victor Starsia

Editor
Richard Day Gore

Library of Congress Control Number: 2008927931

Publisher: LaChance Publishing LLC
              120 Bond Street
              Brooklyn, NY 11217
              www.lachancepublishing.com

Distributor: Independent Publishers Group
              814 North Franklin Street
              Chicago, IL 60610
              www.ipgbook.com

This book is available at special discounts for bulk purchases for sales promotions or premiums. Special editions, including personalized covers, excerpts of existing books, and corporate imprints, can be created in large quantities for special needs. For more information, write to LaChance Publishing, 120 Bond Street, New York, NY 11217 or email info@lachancepublishing.com.

All things have a beginning, although the journey from beginning to end is not always clear and straightforward. While work on *Voices Of* began just a short time ago, the seeds were planted long ago by beloved sources. This book is dedicated to Gennie, Larry and Denise, who in the face of all things good and bad gave courage and support in excess. But especially to Richard, who taught us by the way he lived his life that anything is possible given enough time, hard work and love.

Contents

Part I: Learning

Part II: Commitment

Part III: Compassion

Part IV: Patience

Part V: Forgiveness

Part VI: Humor

Foreword

The New Frontier of Caregiving

Barry Katz

According to a study by the National Family Caregivers Association (NFCA) and the National Alliance for Caregiving (NAC), there are more than 50 million people in the United States caring for loved ones 18 years of age or older. And there are at least another 10 million caring for loved ones with special needs, younger than 18. However staggering these numbers might sound, it appears to be only the tip of the iceberg, as it hardly factors in the impending onslaught of care that the baby-boomer generation will require.

In generations past, most caregiving responsibilities fell to family members who lived in close proximity to their family or friend in need. Today we are seeing a very different picture. Family members are often separated not only by miles, but by states. As a result, the paradigm of caregiving has begun to shift towards one's expanded "circles of community." These circles can encompass family, neighbors, friends, work colleagues and fellow congregants. We are witnessing the coming together of caregiving communities in which all members can reach out and assist in a coordinated manner, regardless of where they are located.

While there is an ever-widening range of websites to visit that are loaded with helpful information about what to expect with regards to caregiving, no practical application or tool had been available to actually help with the caregiving process. Thus the idea for Lotsa Helping Hands was born. Partnered with dozens of leading national nonprofit organizations, Lotsa Helping Hands allows a friend or family member to create a private community where "circles of community," regardless of where its members live, can come together as one unified caregiving group. With more than 10,000 communities created to date, Lotsa Helping Hands has become the cornerstone of new caregiving initiatives for all of these great organizations. This free-of-charge service seamlessly combines the organizational efforts necessary to provide for meals, rides, childcare assistance and activities of daily living (ADL's) with the ability of its members to communicate and provide a variety of timely status updates, blogs, resources, vital information, photo galleries and special sections in which stories and fond memories can be shared by all. In essence, it is a fully functioning caregiving community.

When my wife, Carole Singer, succumbed to her four-year, non-stop battle with ovarian cancer (and I began to think clearly again), it became very evident that there had to be a better way of organizing and coordinating the caregiving process. We had spent far too much time returning phone calls that repeated the same news. We had all too often come home to more than one prepared meal sitting on the front stoop. And we could never quite find the right answer to the popular and constant question, "What can I do to help?"

My experiences with caregiving tell me that in fact most people want very much to lend a helping hand during a time of crisis and illness and often just don't know what to do. They fear becoming intrusive and ultimately part of the problem, rather than seeing themselves as part of the solution. Empowering the ability to communicate, coordinate and organize turns out to be a solution that presents itself as a complete win-win scenario; primary caregivers and their helpers feel better because they can give clear direction as to what is needed, get some needed respite, and overall do not feel like a burden to the process. At the same time, care receivers can also feel good because they no longer have to constantly ask for help, and know in their hearts that when someone in the community signs up to help, it is because they really want to.

This caregiving paradigm shift ultimately begins with communication. Stories need to be told, shared and passed down through the generations. In *Voices of Caregiving*, people from all walks of life share their most intimate stories of how the act of caregiving has transformed the way they view and understand their loved ones, share their joys and fears, and ultimately strengthen the bonds of their relationships. These important stories serve to tear down the walls of isolation that often accompany the rigors of day-to-day caregiving. The common thread throughout the book is that communication, on all levels, contains powerful healing powers. *Voices of Caregiving* will serve as an integral part of a blueprint for the new frontier of caregiving.

Barry Katz is the co-founder and President of Lotsa Helping Hands, a free-of-charge caregiving coordination web service that enables teams of caregivers ("circles of community") to organize and automate the process of caring for loved ones in times of crisis. Lotsa Helping Hands is the recipient of *Today's Caregiver* magazine's 2008 Caregiver Friendly Award.

Prior to founding Lotsa Helping Hands, Mr. Katz co-founded Xevo Corporation, a company that enabled global telecommunications providers to deliver remotely hosted application services over the Internet, and The Career Group LTD, a technology recruiting company that specialized in the staffing and growth planning for start-up technology companies.

Foreword

America's New First Responder: Prisoners of Love Today, Sacred Heroes Tomorrow

James Huysman, Psy.D., LCSW

We are all inspired by the incredible stories of handicapped people who write novels with their toes, cancer victims who run marathons for cancer research, and bereaved parents who set up memorial funds for their lost children. How much easier is it for most of us to be small heroes simply by taking responsibility for our daily lives and transcending our ordinary obstacles?

—*Danah Zohar*

If the needs of 50 million people in this country were being ignored, couldn't we expect a firestorm of protest from every quarter, particularly from those whose needs were being swept under the carpet? But that is exactly what is happening in the United States today to its caregiver population, and hardly a word about it is heard.

The caregivers whose stories you read about throughout this wonderful book are impacted mind, body and soul each and every day by the physical, emotional and psychological toll of giving care to their loved ones. They are challenged by their situation as much as or more than any group receiving the rapt attention of the media. But caregiving is not a sexy, "ratings grabbing" topic that gets the media excited. As the Executive Director and co-founder of the Leeza Gibbons Memory Foundation, an organization advocating for the needs of caregivers, and as one who prides himself on working effectively with the media, I have experienced this disinterest since our founding.

We think it is time to change this sad fact.

For too long, caregiving has been burdened by such negative descriptions as "martyr," "victim," "obligation" and "sacrifice." To the uninformed, caregiving is associated with *codependency*, a mental health challenge in which someone exhibits too much, and often inappropriate, caring for other people's struggles, often enabling bad behavior (e.g., excessive drinking) in the one being cared for. And make no mistake that caregiving can and does trigger "codependency" in many. These associations cause caregivers to avoid being labeled a "caregiver" and, as a result, they fail to take steps to seek help for themselves. The caregivers in this country have truly become "prisoners of love."

I use the phrase "prisoner of love" because our culture often sees caregiving as an obligation. Most believe that if you love someone, then you need to sacrifice for him or her no matter what it takes. Sacrifice is expected. Putting another's needs before one's own is expected. But when a caregiver puts a loved one's *health* ahead of his or her own, the sacrifice can be great: of the mind, body and soul. In the name of love, even death can ensue. In fact, in our practice we are seeing more and more caregivers dying before those receiving their care. The devastating toll that caregiving can inflict on the caregiver often means that no one is left to care for the person who needed care in the first place.

That is why we would like to ask America to reconsider how it perceives the caregiver.

In addition to being a psychologist, I am a certified Compassion Fatigue Therapist. Compassion Fatigue is a state experienced by those helping people in distress; it is an extreme state of tension and a preoccupation with the suffering of those being helped to the degree that it traumatizes the helper, causing deep physical, spiritual and emotional exhaustion and pain. In my role as a compassion fatigue therapist, I work with First Responders: community heroes such as policemen, firemen, emergency medical technicians, clergy members, nurses, therapists and others.

Working daily with people in need, they are vulnerable to anxiety, sleep disturbance, depression, cynicism, anger and irritability, and difficulty separating their work from their personal life. It is the emotional residue of exposure to the suffering of others. Compassion fatigue occurs when professionals and lay people alike become emotionally drained by the pain and trauma of their patients and families. The helpers still care and want to help, but they do not have the emotional energy to do so. They suffer their own secondary traumatic stress and begin to seem detached and "burned out."

If you are a caregiver or work with caregivers, does all this sound familiar? You see, it becomes more and more evident that the caregiver's challenges mirror those of the traditional first responder. In fact, like the first responders we know and respect, few would doubt that caregivers often find themselves, figuratively, running into their family's burning homes while other members of the family are running out. Thus, caregivers are also first responders, Family First Responders™ as we call them at the Leeza Gibbons Memory Foundation.

The word "caregiver" does less to get people's attention than referring to the person as a Family First Responder. We as a society would be better served by thinking of and depicting these individuals not as "caregivers," a term that conjures up visions of Mother Teresa and martyrdom, but as first responders. In fact, like our country's first responders, Family First Responders are American heroes.

When Leeza and I began to refer to caregivers as Family First Responders, we saw the caregivers that came to Leeza's Place, and the media that were reporting on them, perk up, take notice and be more inclined to listen. We also found that caregivers felt better about themselves. Our caregivers are relieved that they can be proud of what they do, that it can bring them to a place of being honored rather than to a place of shame and stigma.

We at the Leeza Gibbons Memory Foundation have identified a population over 50 million strong that we believe either suffer from compassion fatigue or are at risk to suffer it. And we believe that it is a compelling national story, a powerful health story and a sacred heroic story that needs to be told and honored by all.

America and American corporations will reap the benefits of lower healthcare costs and increased productivity as more caregivers receive treatment for compassion fatigue. Employees who are caregivers experience decreased efficiency, diminished initiative, reduced interest in work, depleted ability to work under stress, difficulty concentrating, and increased irritation with coworkers. This often leads to the increased use of tranquilizers, alcohol and cigarettes. Recognizing the caregiver as a first responder will contribute to the growth in the self-esteem of a population that desperately needs it. It will lead to caregivers proudly identifying themselves as caregivers and it will allow these heroes to stand up for themselves and be noticed, by their families, their communities and their country.

So what does this mean for the future? The number of Family First Responders will grow geometrically as the baby boomers age; by 2020, we expect their ranks to grow to some 80 million. If they suffer from burnout and compassion fatigue, their immunological systems will be compromised and medical costs will skyrocket. New perspectives and prevention models such as are to be found at Leeza's Place will be vitally needed to deal with this potential healthcare crisis. The future is ominous if we do not look at caregivers in a different light and if caregivers do not see themselves in a different light.

The future health of our country demands that we recognize caregivers as Family First Responders, to see them as professionals taking care of themselves and who see their journey as heroic, not victimizing. We hope that our caregivers will eventually embrace the idea of caregiving as heroic work. At Leeza's Place, we honor their stories, bear witness to their heroism and walk alongside them with sacred recognition and respect. As caregivers find their way to a Leeza's Place, we hope they realize that the opportunity to give to others is a blessing. When they become proud of their role, they become the model of emotional experience for many others.

———————————

Dr. James Huysman is the co-founder and Executive Director of the Leeza Gibbons Memory Foundation, a nonprofit organization dedicated to the education and empowerment of caregivers and their family members who suffer from long-term memory disorders. He is a psychologist, board-certified therapist in clinical social work, crisis interventionist and nationally certified addictions professional. His varied career has included a responsive advocacy, client care and progressive health services development. The recipient of a doctorate in psychology from the Southern California School of Professional Studies and a master's degree in social work from Barry University, he has developed national programs, and served as a clinical consultant and as an officer for a large number of national hospitals and independent psychiatric and addictions centers.

Foreword

The Caregiving Crisis in America

Laura Bauer Granberry, MPA

The United States is in the midst of a significant and growing caregiving crisis. Although people are living longer, the number of family members available to provide care has grown smaller, and we are facing a critical shortage of direct care workers as well. About 1.4 million older Americans live in nursing homes, nearly 6 million receive care at home, and significant numbers go completely without the help they need. The goal of the Rosalynn Carter Institute for Caregiving (RCI) is to increase the quality of long-term, home and community-based care in America. We believe there must be a fundamental shift in how our nation values caregiving and caregivers: all sectors of society must come together in new ways to develop solutions. There are a number of strategies that must be undertaken if we are to make real progress in achieving this goal.

One strategy is to increase the number of *evidence-based caregiver programs* operating around the country. Evidence-based programs are those that have been proven to be effective by rigorous scientific evaluation and that are strongly linked to desirable outcomes, such as reductions in caregivers' depressive symptoms and increases in measures of coping. An example of an existing evidence-based caregiver program is the New York University Caregiver Intervention (NYUCI), developed some 20 years ago by Dr. Mary Mittelman. A counseling and support intervention program for spouse caregivers, NYUCI is intended to improve the well-being of caregivers and delay the nursing home placement of patients with Alzheimer's disease. The program aims to help spouse caregivers mobilize their social support network and better adapt to their caregiving role. Although not widely known outside the research community, many other interventions with proven positive outcomes for caregivers—programs that really help caregivers—have already been developed.

The problem is that most have not been translated into actual programs that can be delivered at the community level. There are many reasons for this research/practice gap. Lack of knowledge and lack of financial support from funding agencies are major barriers. Some programs do not offer training opportunities and may not have developed training materials that can be used by others. Many agencies tend to think that getting evidence-based programs up and running is difficult and time-consuming. As a result, families continue to be underserved and do not receive proven strategies. But there is hope! Many evidence-based caregiver interventions (several still in the research phase) have been identified, some of which are already in use and some of which are currently being successfully translated into practice in community settings.

A second critical strategy is to improve quality in workforce development. Fewer and fewer individuals are seeking employment in caregiving occupations and turnover for those in the field is high for many reasons—low wages, bad working conditions, lack of fringe benefits, the physical and emotional strains of the job, and the lack of career ladder advancement are just a few. Many people are not aware of the fact that family caregivers in the United States provide approximately $307 *billion* dollars of unpaid care each year. If these caregivers are not properly supported in that role, they may suffer their own negative emotional and/or physical consequences, leaving them unable to continue to provide care for their loved ones. Should this happen on a large scale, there would simply not be enough hospital or nursing home beds or paid caregivers in the workforce to handle the shortfall.

A third strategy is to increase both public awareness of the dimensions of quality care and the advocacy needed to to achieve them. We believe that quality long-term care in the community should be:

- **Safe**—avoiding injuries to care-receivers (and caregivers) from the care that is intended to help them.

- **Effective**—providing services based on scientific knowledge to all who could benefit and refraining from providing services to those not likely to benefit.

- **Personalized**—providing care that is respectful of and responsive to individual care-receiver (and caregiver) preferences, needs and values and ensuring that care-receiver (and caregiver) values guide all clinical decisions.

- **Timely**—reducing waits and harmful delays for both those who receive and those who give care.

- **Efficient**—avoiding waste, including waste of equipment, supplies, ideas and energy.

- **Equitable**—providing care that does not vary in quality because of personal characteristics such as gender, ethnicity, geographic location and socioeconomic status.

- **Balanced**—providing care that is integrated into the daily life of care-receiver and caregiver and that facilitates self-determination and a rich life in the community.

- **Shared**—providing adequate support, respite and assistance to family caregivers so that the objective burdens of care, including financial and time-related burdens, are shared as much as possible between professional caregivers, family caregivers and others in the community.

- **Collaborative**—integrating the work of family, professional caregivers and the community in a way that maximizes their unique contributions, skills and knowledge.

- **Developmental**—providing a range of services and supports in a manner that facilitates development, learning and the achievement of personal goals for the care-receiver and members of the long-term care team.*

In collaboration with many other organizations, agencies and individuals, the RCI believes that positive gains are being made in all of these areas. I welcome you to log onto our website (www.RosalynnCarter.org) for updates on what is happening in the field. As Mrs. Carter often states, "There are only four kinds of people in the world: those who have been caregivers, those who currently are caregivers, those who will be caregivers, and those who will need caregivers." As a result, quality care should be *everyone's* concern.

Laura Bauer Granberry is the Director of National Initiatives for the Rosalynn Carter Institute for Caregiving, an organization created in 1987 on the campus of Georgia Southwestern State University in honor of former First Lady Rosalynn Carter, a GSW alumna. RCI seeks to establish local, state and national partnerships committed to building quality long-term, home and community-based services and to provide greater recognition and support for America's professional and family caregivers. Its main focus is supporting individuals and caregivers coping with chronic illness and disability across their life spans. She is the co-author of two of the RCI signature training programs, *Caring for You, Caring for Me—Education and Support for Family and Professional Caregivers, 2nd Edition* and *Caring and Competent Caregivers: Professionals Helping Families.*

---

*Birkel, Richard C., "Defining Quality Care in Long-Term, Home and Community Settings."

Introduction
The Healing Project
Debra LaChance

I wanted to ask the people around me, "Would you please raise your hand if you feel as isolated as I do?" Walking the busy streets of Manhattan on a beautiful sunny day, I was surrounded by people but I'd never felt so alone. Just minutes before, my doctors had broken the news to me that I had a particularly aggressive form of breast cancer.

Since moving to New York from a small town in Rhode Island, I'd had my share of ups and downs but had always risen to the challenges that living and working in New York can bring. But on this summer afternoon, I felt as if the world was suddenly rushing past me while I seemed to be moving in slow motion; I was completely alone.

After recovering from the initial shock I found that one of the first things I almost automatically began to look for, besides doctors, was a sense of connection. I needed to hear from other people who had gone through what I was experiencing, who truly understood what it meant and who might be able to help. I wasn't ready for a regular support group, and with surgery and treatment looming, I simply didn't have the time. But I am an avid reader, and I assumed that finding the personal stories of those who had gone through this ordeal before me would be relatively easy. But there seemed to be a vacuum; almost nothing. Where were the real people to talk to? Where was the literature that wasn't just about the hardcore science of the disease, but about how to cope?

There was one book that gave me great solace, *Just Get Me Through This* by Deborah Cohen and Robert A. Gelfand. It was more of a personal story, rather than a clinical one, and it created in me a desire for more stories that get to the heart of the emotional experience, that help the reader through it. I knew there must be countless others out there who needed to tell their stories—and to hear the stories of others as well. I decided that part of my own, ongoing healing process would be to find a way to bring people like me together, to create some kind of forum where these real stories could be shared.

Over time my vision of community crystallized and The Healing Project was born. I'd already realized that having access to the real stories of real people would make the journey through breast cancer much easier to endure. My thoughts kept returning to that walk through Manhattan after I'd heard my diagnosis and that feeling of terrible loneliness. As sympathetic as friends and loved ones could be, I felt that no one could truly understand this journey except someone who had made it before. I was convinced that getting and giving courage, comfort, and strength were as important as good medical care, and I became determined to help build a community for people like me who were undergoing the terribly isolating experience of dealing with a life-threatening or chronic disease. This would be The Healing Project's mission: to become a bridge across which people can make those all-important emotional connections.

And those are the people I want to help me build The Healing Project community. I began to develop The Healing Project as a place where people can contribute funds for research, time for connecting with others, and most of all, a place to share their stories. Since then, The Healing Project has been collecting stories by those touched by illness or diseases for books like this one: books that inspire and inform for the road ahead and impart a sense of community for those caught up in dealing with the moment. When you're sick or afraid, it's a godsend to know that there are others who understand. These books are meant to be a companion for patients, their friends, and families, an oasis where they can find strength in shared experiences.

In addition to the books, we're also working on other initiatives through The Healing Project, including Voices Who Care, a "virtual support group" which will allow family and friends to connect with others in real time. I don't want anyone to have to feel the way I did the day of my diagnosis when I was walking through the city alone and afraid. There's so much strength in others—you just have to find them.

When you are dealing with disease, you have to be ready to chart a new course, for the rest of your life, no matter what the outcome. And it helps to see that others are busy charting their own courses along with you. That's what these stories are all about. Reading these amazing contributions to the *Voices Of* series convinces me that I don't really have a uniquely remarkable story at all.

The truth is everyone does.

Debra LaChance is the creator and founder of The Healing Project.

The Healing Project

Individuals diagnosed with life-threatening or chronic, debilitating illnesses face countless physical, emotional, social, spiritual, and financial challenges during their treatment and throughout their lives. The support of family members, friends, and the community at large is essential to their successful recovery and their quality of life and access to accurate and current information about their illnesses enables patients and their caregivers to make informed decisions about treatment and post-treatment care. Founded in 2005 by Debra LaChance, The Healing Project is dedicated to promoting the health and well-being of these individuals, developing resources to enhance their quality of life, and supporting the family members and friends who care for them. For more information about The Healing Project and its programs, please visit our website at www.thehealingproject.org.

Acknowledgments

This book would not have been possible without the selfless dedication of many people giving freely of their valuable time and expertise. We'd particularly like to thank Theresa Russell, Alice Bergmann and Amy Shore for their work reaching out to the people and organizations making so many contributions to this book; Melissa Marr for her invaluable assistance, insights and opinions; Drs. James Huysman, Rosemary Laird and Cynthia Pan, together with Barry Katz, Laura Bauer Granberry and Ooi-Thye Chong, for sharing their professional expertise; and to the many, many people who submitted their stories to us, for their courage, their generosity and their humanity.

Part I
Learning

… comes in many forms for the caregiver,
from medical knowledge to new self-awareness.

Why Me?

Dan Gordon

The thing about becoming a caregiver is that you don't have any say in the matter. It's just something that falls to you when something bad happens to someone close. When my wife, Judy, was diagnosed with cancer, I became the designated caregiver. Nobody asked; it was just presumed. No matter that it was not a role I had aspired to, nor was it something I felt I would be any good at. And, of course, the timing was terrible. In fact, it was probably the one thing in the world I least wanted—except, of course, Judy having cancer. Oops. Right at the start, that's one of the problems with being a caregiver—you can't whine about it without sounding like a jerk.

I mean it's not like I ever considered not taking on the responsibility. After all, it concerned Judy, and Judy and I had been an item for almost forty years. So I was going to do it—it's just that I first had to indulge in a little woe-is-me. That would have to be done in the privacy of my own thoughts, which is right where I went once the initial chaos caused by the diagnosis subsided. There I started mentally going over everything that was wrong with being stuck in such a position. Then, when I tired of wallowing around in that quagmire, I started listing out exactly what being a caregiver would entail. I wanted to prepare Judy ahead of time for all the ways I would not be of any value to her when she needed me the most. It was important that we both knew what to reasonably expect from me, and more important, what not to expect, so other arrangements could be made.

From observing others take on the role, mostly in movies, I divided caregiving into three basic parts. The first was simply being present, always being around when a warm body was needed. I had no problem with that; attendance had always been one of my best subjects. As an additional benefit, caregiving gave me a legitimate reason to play fast and loose with my schedule at work.

The second involved relieving Judy of various everyday, mundane chores that might become overwhelming. I felt I already did more than my fair share of stuff around the house, but I supposed I could add paying the bills and an occasional vacuuming to the list. So the first two caregiving chores didn't seem overly difficult; they actually looked very doable.

The third part, however, appeared daunting. It had to do with being able to speak the words of comfort and support that would help her get through the rough times. The problem is that I've always been more of the strong silent type, a true believer in actions speaking louder than words. So I never was much of a talker. Small talk and comforting words were foreign to me, yet they were just what was needed and expected. They would help fill the slow-passing time, provide the necessary distractions from moments of acute discomfort, and counteract the frightening episodes of feeling unable to cope any longer. While I understand the value of this, I simply was not very skilled at it. Whenever I tried my hand at it, it sounded like I was forcing myself through a most unpleasant task, which is just what was occurring. My saying "there, there, it'll be all right" sounded like I had a terminal case of stage fright, making the audience more likely to wince at my discomfort than find any relief for theirs. Part of the problem is my need to truly believe in what I'm saying. I can't say things like, "You'll be right as rain in no time" unless I know for certain that that will be the ultimate result. But, despite these reservations, I decided that it was something I could do. I would try to provide all the comfort and support Judy needed.

Except things don't always turn out well just because you've decided they will. What I found out early, and then often, was that my simplistic concept of caregiving was not so much inaccurate as it was inadequate. It proved to be a lot more than just dusting the shelves when Judy didn't feel up to it. In fact, my model fell apart during our initial meeting with the surgeon, the first doctor we saw after the diagnosis. She gave us three treatment options: lumpectomy followed by seven weeks of radiation, mastectomy, or mastectomy with reconstructive surgery. As we sat and listened to these options, I already knew the answer. With all our history together, Judy and I had grown to know how each other thought, and in this situation I knew Judy would choose the least invasive treatment, the one that would leave the fewest memories of ever having had breast cancer. I almost spoke for her to tell the doctor it would be door number one, lumpectomy and radiation. But Judy spoke first and selected door number three, mastectomy with reconstruction. Not only radical and invasive, but the one that included plastic surgery and eight weeks recovery time. I stared at her in disbelief.

Discussing it later, I learned that even forty years together did not make me privy to all her cranial nooks and crannies. She told me that her dread of cancer was such that the minimalist countermeasure of minor surgery and radiation would not leave her feeling safe. Only the most drastic measures would give her the peace of mind that comes from knowing she had done all she could to get rid of the disease and prevent its recurrence. As she was explaining that to me, I prepared my counter-argument, which I knew would convince her that she was wrong and that I knew what was best. "I have the clearer head right now," I silently rehearsed my rebuttal. "I'm not as emotionally mixed-up right now, because it's not happening to my body."

When I heard those words of advice I was about to give, I started envisioning how I would respond if it was, in fact, happening to my body. I would not want somebody else's version of "what's right" imposed on me. It would be my body, and my decision. All I would want from my caregiver, or anyone else, was support— not debate. So when the time came to respond to Judy's explanation of her decision, all I wanted to know was that she clearly understood the implications of each option, and that she was certain about her choice. She did, and she was, and so I gave her my complete support, choosing not to cast any doubt onto the decision she had obviously taken great care in making. But it was not easy for me to bite my tongue. I was used to being a lawgiver, not a caregiver. I had life pretty well figured out and knew what was right for me, and for everyone else as well. But I was beginning to understand that being a caregiver overruled the certain wisdom of the know-it-all. I had to open up to other versions of "what's right" even if I was sure they were wrong.

Of course, making that adjustment was not the end of it. My choosing to suppress my opinions on Judy's treatment did not mean everyone else would suppress theirs. This became more of an issue when Judy's cancer proved more aggressive than first thought and the treatment plan expanded to include a rigorous regimen of chemotherapy after a mastectomy without reconstructive surgery. The extended treatment, and the devastating effects chemo had on her, forced us to call more and more upon family, friends, and professionals to assist in caring for her. The upshot of going public in this way forced me, as caregiver, into a role not unlike a presidential press secretary. I was the one everyone counted on for the latest info, and spin, on how she was doing. Being on the frontline like that was a position my introverted nature was ill-suited for. I was the person to whom many people voiced their opinions on what Judy's treatment should and should not include. Apparently, there are a lot of people out there, like me, who know "what's right" for everyone. Having, with some difficulty, resolved that issue for myself, I now had to resolve it over and over again. I needed to constantly remind myself that those who did speak their mind to me did so with Judy's best interests at heart, and because they were helping out in other ways, it was not appropriate for me to get testy with them. But they, and their recommendations, did need to be dealt with and reflected upon. So with each new suggestion, I found myself revisiting the treatment decisions we had already made. Each time I re-wondered if we had chosen the best option. What if we chose wrong? What if we had missed something else, something more likely to succeed? Should I have been more assertive in directing her treatment? My once-simple caregiving model was becoming more complex with each passing event.

And in that year following the diagnosis, very little time passed between events. Just getting used to riding the roller coaster of good news and bad news, good days and bad days, was a major achievement. Learning to expect the unexpected became neces-- sary, as did developing an artificial equanimity in responding to all that transpired. Not getting too hopeful when things were going well, or too despairing when things went bad, were necessary for being ready to handle the next inevitable rise or fall of the jour- ney. Caregiving turned out to be a lot about acting nonchalant while the roller coaster went through its paces.

In the end, the biggest change to my concept of caregiving was not about what I had to do as a caregiver, but how I became one. Facing a life-altering situation led to a lot of reflection and in doing so I realized that the role of caregiver was not suddenly thrust upon me by Judy's diagnosis. Instead, becoming a caregiver was something I had signed up for way back when Judy and I decided to spend the rest of our lives together. We may not have thought about it in specific terms, but when we chose to live and grow old together we were tacitly acknowledging that somewhere along the way things might not be so happily ever after. Things would happen to us. The longer we were together, the more likely life would challenge us. No one remains unscathed, just as no one gets out alive. So caregiver was just another one of the inevitable roles I chose to take on when we formed our company. Along with friend, lover, parent, provider, and unconditional supporter, I agreed to be a caregiver. I did it as well as I could, and probably could have done it better. But I could not imagine not doing it. And while I found it difficult, and occasionally even scary, I never found it draining. I was honored to do it, and grateful for the opportunity. I wouldn't have it any other way.

Dan Gordon has worked as a mental health caseworker, management consultant, and community college instructor, but most of his career has been spent in the retail arena. He writes for pleasure and has co-authored with his wife *The Heroics of Falling Apart: One Couple's Breast Cancer Journey*. He lives with his family in Denver.

Palliative Care and Hospice

Cynthia X. Pan, MD

One unanticipated result of the advances made in healthcare during the past century has been the emergence of chronic illness as the leading cause of death. At the same time, the enhanced ability to significantly extend life for patients with chronic diseases has blurred the boundary between curable illnesses and illnesses that inevitably result in death. As a result, over the course of the 20th century, Western society has increasingly attributed near-miraculous powers to medical science—and increasingly avoided the subject of death. Many patients and physicians came to regard the prolongation of life and the cure of disease as the fundamental and exclusive goals of modern medicine. Viewed from this perspective, death is considered to be a medical failure.

Recent decades, however, have seen a growing recognition that this view is unrealistic and potentially harmful. This recognition has supported the emergence of the field of *palliative care*. Unlike curative care, which focuses on the disease process, palliative care focuses on the patient, striving to minimize the patient's burden and maximize the patient's quality of life. It also focuses on the caregiver, recognizing that the caregiver suffers alongside the patient but is often overlooked, and that no plan of care for a seriously ill patient can succeed without a dedicated caregiver.

Palliative care is a discipline that openly acknowledges dying as part of living and does not consider death an enemy. In this way, palliative care encourages open and honest discussions about the patient's illness, concerns, worries, hopes, and legacies. It also encourages the use of hospice services when the patient is considered terminally ill, since hospice can provide comprehensive health benefits and a financial safety net for the patient and the family. Palliative care and hospice both consider the patient and the caregiver as a single unit of care, acknowledging the critical role of the caregiver during times of serious or terminal illness.

Death and Dying in the United States

Most people in this country can now expect to die in old age. Of the over 2 million deaths per year in the United States, an estimated 73% occur in persons 65 years of age or older. In 2008, the estimated life expectancy at birth reached 78.2 years, compared with less than 50 years in 1900. The median age of death in the United States is 78; of persons who survive to 65 years of age, median age at death is in the 80's. Persons 65 years of age or older constitute an increasingly large proportion of the United States population: in 1999, persons 65 years of age or older accounted for about 13% of the population and this proportion is projected to rise to 20% by the year 2030. Persons 85 years of age or older constitute the most rapidly growing segment. The three leading causes of death in adults in the United States in 2006 were heart disease, *malignant neoplasm* (cancer), and stroke. *Chronic obstructive pulmonary disease* (COPD), pneumonia, and accidents each accounted for less than 10% of all deaths. Most adult deaths in the United States occur in hospitals (56%), followed by deaths occurring at home (21%), in nursing homes (19%), and in other settings (4%). These statistics vary substantially according to geographic location, primarily because of regional variations in hospital, hospice, and nursing home bed supply.

The elderly population is extremely heterogeneous, varying in socioeconomic status, educational level, and cultural and ethnic background. This diversity is likely to increase in the coming years. For example, African Americans 65 years of age and older numbered 2.5 million in 1990 (constituting 8% of the population of persons older than 65 years), and their number is expected to more than triple, to 8.4 million (or 10.5% of that population), by 2030. Similarly, there were approximately 1.1 million Hispanic elderly persons in 1990 (3.5% of the population of persons older than 65 years), but by 2030 this number will skyrocket to 12.5 million (15.6% of that group). The number and percentage of Asian elderly are ever increasing as well.

Compared with the current elderly population, elderly baby boomers will be far more knowledgeable about healthcare and far more demanding of healthcare providers. Their expectations are likely to lead them to challenge the health care profession to deliver high quality end-of-life care tailored to patients' individual needs and to provide that care in a culturally sensitive manner.

Although most deaths occur in the elderly, people can become critically ill at any point in their lives and can die at any age. In fact, the persons whose cases formed the basis for establishing important precedents for ethical and legal decisions related to death and dying were young adults: 26-year-old Nancy Cruzan in Missouri, whose case involved the issue of artificial feeding of patients in a persistent vegetative state; and 21-year-old Karen Ann Quinlan of New Jersey, whose case involved the withdrawal of artificial ventilation (breathing machine) from patients in a persistent vegetative state. Most recently, the case of Terri Schiavo in Florida shook the nation, prompting many people to seriously think about making their wishes about the end of life known before a serious illness strikes. Thus, despite these statistics, people can become seriously ill and die at any age. Hospice and palliative care provide services for people with serious or terminal illnesses, regardless of age.

(continued on page 40)

My Own Sixth Sense

Toni Weingarten

When I try to describe my work as a hospital chaplain, I sometimes fall back on the line from the film *The Sixth Sense*: "I see dead people."

Death and dying are a natural part of life, yet most of us are far removed from them; I know I was. The only dead person I'd ever seen was my father. So my time at the hospital has shown me that death and dying come in as many forms as there are people and lifestyles. As someone told us in a hospital lecture on dying, "people pretty much die as they lived." People with dysfunctional families often die amidst tumult: at times the family members are estranged and the remaining parent and adult children may hurl angry words at one another over the lifeless corpse as we hospital chaplains try to offer some form of comfort or coming together amidst the flying barbs. We leave these encounters shaking our heads in disbelief at the discord amidst the family members in both life and in death.

Then there are the moments such as the one I recently witnessed.

I received a call to be with a family that had just removed their mother from mechanical life support. I felt nervous approaching their room and when I entered I saw two adult men and one woman, all in tears, around the bed of their unconscious mother. The daughter tenderly stroked her mother's forehead, and the sons each held one of her hands, which they caressed between bending to plant it with a kiss.

I walked in and put my hand on the daughter's shoulder, gently rubbing it in acknowledgment of her sorrow.

"Hi, I'm Toni, one of the chaplains. How are you holding up?"

One of the brothers looked up and said, "We're okay. She's getting what she wants. She wouldn't have wanted to go to a nursing home"

"Yeah," chimed in the other brother. "But she wouldn't want a lot of fuss from us right now."

And then he looked at his mother, her face somewhat contorted as she struggled for breath without assist from a machine, and he said, "But we're getting the last word, Mom. We're making a fuss over you!"

His brother and sister broke into smiles and laughed. "Yeah, she likes things simple but we're treating her special now."

There was so much love in the room that it overshadowed the pain of her dying. The camaraderie and teasing that existed in the family in life continued in death. The siblings proceeded to show me pictures of their mother in better days, and recounted how she had enjoyed their last family dinner and then, the next day, had a stroke and now here she was. I said some words and prayers of comfort and left them to hold vigil for their mother, who died a few hours later. And I was left with the afterglow of their love, not the pain of their loss.

The first time I assisted a family in losing a parent, I put on a long face since I thought that was expected of me as a chaplain—to share, and feel, the family's pain. My supervisor, a longtime chaplain, later took me aside and told me not to do that.

"You're there to be a centering force for them, not to take on their pain."

I was taken aback, as I thought I'd appear unfeeling if I didn't look as though I, too, suffered along with them. Over time, I've come to see the wisdom of my supervisor's words.

The time both before and after the death of a loved one is so intense that people experience the full spectrum of emotions from laughter to grief, from joy to despair; it is as if people are transported to a special realm where stages of life overlap and the regular boundaries separating life events melt away, leaving people streaking across decades and back again in just a few minutes. As chaplain, I serve as their witness, their anchor, one grounded in the present to bring them back to this moment.

So where is God in all this?

Well, it is all about Love and God is in the Love. He is in the gratitude the dying feel for the good they've had in life, and that their loved ones feel for the memories in knowing and loving them. God is in the tenderness the children of a dying parent show at the parent's bedside. He is in the graciousness the families offer me, a stranger who appears in their most difficult moments. Amidst their own pain, they treat me with kindness. God is in how we treat one another in life and in death.

When I say, "I see dead people," I see much more than that. I see the reflection of God in the actions of people made in God's image. In you, I see the divine. And I hope I will show you the same when you come to comfort me.

Toni Weingarten lives near San Francisco where she works as a hospital chaplain and writes on issues of religion and faith. Her writing has appeared in *The New York Times*, *The Christian Science Monitor*, *Newsweek* magazine and others. Visit her website at www.toniweingarten.com.

Mom Had Alzheimer's
Ruth A. Brandwein

How does one start to talk about the disappearance of a mother? Not her physical disappearance, but the gradual disappearance of her personality, her personhood.

When it began, I went into denial. It was after my father died that my sister and I noticed changes in her behavior, but I, a professional social worker, attributed it to the depression that is common after the death of a lifetime companion. My sister suspected otherwise.

Mom began to be paranoid, imagining her neighbors breaking into her home and stealing old clothes from the basement. At first, we wanted to believe her; we knew that sometimes older people's credibility is questioned because of their age. We wanted to give her the respect that she was due. But finally, when she insisted that a neighbor had climbed through the window to steal the electric bill that she couldn't find, we had the doctor assess her condition. She confirmed that Mom was in the early stages of Alzheimer's.

Should we tell her or not? I came up with the idea of asking her if she wanted to be told. One Sunday, during my usual phone call to her, I asked, "Mom, I was just wondering if, God forbid, you should have cancer or Alzheimer's, or something like that, would you want to know?" "Of course I would want to know!" was her clear reply. A month later we had the doctor tell her. She accepted the information, but seemed unable to absorb it.

Soon, we realized it was not safe for her to stay at home alone. But she would not move; she was adamant. "Charlie is here with me," she would say, our father's name bringing tears to our eyes. Both my sister and I had too much respect for her wishes to move her against her will, but she needed help if she was going to stay. I had to fight with her Medicare HMO to allow for a social work assessment: first, I argued that Alzheimer's was, in fact, a medical condition. Then I argued cost efficiency: it would be more expensive if she injured herself and needed to be hospitalized. Finally, they relented.

The social worker sent to assess my mother was a true professional. He addressed his questions to her rather than to us. My mother was resistant to having anyone in the house, even a home care worker for a few hours each day. He said to her, "I know you want to be independent. Sometimes the way to stay as independent as possible is to get the help you need." She liked and trusted him and agreed to have a worker come in five days a week to help prepare meals and oversee her medications. His approach showed consummate skill—showing her respect, treating her with dignity, acknowledging her overwhelming need for autonomy and independence.

But Mom quickly forgot what she had agreed to during the social worker's visit. We hired someone, but Mom kept fighting with her and "firing" her. We kept convincing her to return—by then, Mom would have forgotten she had "fired" her.

The early stages of Alzheimer's are hardest, I believe, on the person suffering from it. The later stages are hardest on the family. As my daughter said later, "It used to be that she'd be OK and then a fog would come down over her. Now, it seems like the fog is there all the time, and sometimes, for just a brief time, it lifts and she seems like Grandma."

After it became apparent that the part-time worker would not work out, we tried putting Mom into an Alzheimer's unit at a well-respected nursing home. However, at that time she was still physically mobile. The unit really did not meet her needs. Most of the residents were in the later stages of the disease and sat fixed in wheelchairs. Mom was enraged. "Get me out of here! These people are crazy! If you don't take me out, I'll leave and walk home." After three days we got her out, and by some miracle we found a kind woman to live with her. This woman was from Tonga, where the elderly are respected. Over the next three years she, her sister, and then a niece cared for Mom at home until she died. Fortunately my parents had saved money over the years, and we gradually cashed in their CDs to pay for Mom's care.

My sister lived nearby and was able to check on Mom daily and arrange for doctors' appointments, purchase medications, and deal with emergencies. Mom was on several medications, for both congestive heart failure and Alzheimer's. She was losing weight and complained of insomnia. Finally, her doctor determined that the medications were no longer helping her and took her off most, even replacing Coumadin, a blood thinner, with aspirin. Amazingly, she slept better and her appetite returned. "Where is my breakfast?" she'd demand of her helper, not remembering that she had eaten breakfast an hour ago. That wonderful woman wouldn't argue with her, but would simply prepare another breakfast.

My sister and I were able to agree on most details about Mom's care, although I must admit that the roles of older and younger sister sometimes got in the way. It is not unusual that during a parent's last years siblings will replay their childhood relationships. I finally became aware that this was happening between us and was able to recognize my "kid" sister as the able, competent adult she now was.

Several hospitalizations over time caused Mom terrible anxiety and she seemed to mentally deteriorate after each one. She was now entering the last stage of Alzheimer's. She no longer recognized us. She had become physically frail, somewhat incontinent, and almost blind. I knew that most frail elderly who get pneumonia and survive it last, on average, only another six months. My sister and I both agreed that if Mom got pneumonia, we would not send her to a hospital. When, at 89, she contracted pneumonia and we told the doctor our wishes, she arranged for hospice care. Mom died four days later, in her own home, surrounded by her family. It was a good death.

So, what have I learned? Even as a professional, my emotions as a daughter often got in the way of my "professionalism." At a time like this, being a daughter, son, or spouse is one's primary role. It's important to recognize this and to get all the help that is available. It is imperative to continue to treat the person with Alzheimer's with respect and to recognize that she is grasping to maintain control of her own life. Don't argue and try to rationally convince that person. At this point, she is not rational. Like small children, sometimes distractions work better.

It helps to maintain a sense of humor. As they say, sometimes you have to laugh to keep from crying. It's also important to keep your sentences simple—complex sentences confuse them. Don't say, "Do you want to go for a walk or do you want to go shopping?" Just ask, "Do you want to go for a walk?" Work to overcome old patterns of dysfunctional behavior among siblings. Let go of whatever old rivalries and grudges that may lie under the surface of these relationships. Working together on behalf of a loved one is paramount.

Finally, what we realized when Mom was in the late stages and couldn't recognize us is that she would respond to human warmth and to touch. She'd say, "I don't know who you are, but I like you." Her rational processes had shut down, but she could still sense the feeling of love and caring. Although the mother I had known gradually disappeared, I still loved the woman she had become. She may not have known my name, but I know she still loved me.

———————

Ruth A. Brandwein is a professor and the former dean of the Stony Brook University School of Social Welfare and is the Director of the school's Social Justice Center.

Ben and the Snow Storm

Kay Cavanaugh

The driving storm that blanketed the narrow mountain roads with snow made for a grueling journey. But my patient Ben was low on his pain medicine and the thought of him sitting in this storm with no one but his loyal old dog Bo kept me from canceling the trip.

I have been a nurse in this Blue Ridge Mountain town for twenty years. Ben, age eighty, was referred to me by his surgeon. Ben was recovering from the removal of a lobe of his right lung. He had decided against chemotherapy or radiation, letting nature take its course. "Doc told me the cancer already spread to my bones," Ben had told me. "Ain't no sense in filling this old body with poison." I had to agree.

Ben lived in an old, dilapidated house perched far up on a mountainside. As the trip wore on I questioned my decision to keep the appointment. My windshield wipers weren't working fast enough to clear the falling snow and I ended up driving with the window down, my arm stretched around to the windshield, trying to brush the icy snow from the glass as I drove. My arm turning numb, I could barely keep ahead of the snow as it distorted my view of the fast-disappearing road. I had been up that mountain 'holler' several times before, but with no road signs for miles and the heavy snowfall it was hard to recognize any familiar reference points on the way to Ben's place.

I drove until the road abruptly ended at an empty, snow-filled field. I gathered the supplies I needed to change his surgical dressing, took a deep breath, and stepped out into at least four feet of packed snow. Barely able to make out anything in the distance, I trudged up the hillside towards Ben's house with the bitterly cold wind biting at my cheeks. The snow filled my boots and my toes were starting to go numb. The wind whipped up the powdery snow, obscuring my view. I tried to remember the symptoms of hypothermia; I was sure being disoriented was one of them, and I began to feel that now.

Another thirty minutes through the blizzard and I reached a house that was unrecognizable in the drifts, promising myself that if Ben didn't live there I was going to give nursing care to whoever did. I stamped my numb and stinging feet on the wooden porch and brushed off the rest of the snow from my boots with a tattered old broom that was leaning against the door.

I pounded on the door. "Ben, it's your nurse," I called. Ben responded, "Come in out of that weather, darling."

I stepped inside and Bo greeted me by slamming his large, bedraggled hindquarter against my legs, almost knocking me off my feet. The smell of burning wood from Ben's black potbellied stove filled my dripping nose. After the bitter chill outside it was hot, almost suffocating, in the little house.

Ben lived out his life in two tiny rooms. The parlor was furnished with a day bed, a rocking chair, the wood burning stove and two kerosene lamps, with two windows covered by pumpkin-colored plastic curtains. Several handmade quilts I had given him lay on the day bed. The second room, even smaller than the first, had an undersized sink and a small icebox that used ice blocks to keep his food cold. A shelf of warped plywood held his food supplies along with two cracked brown ceramic plates, two battered aluminum pots, one black metal skillet and a few assorted utensils. On the wall of the parlor facing his chair was the room's only decoration:

an old picture of his parents on their wedding day, yellowed with age and set in an old brass frame. The wooden floors were old, cracked and uneven.

Soon the room felt deliciously warm and the snow in my hair and on my eyelashes started to melt. Ben looked me over and said in the voice of a father telling his young one what to do, "Take them boots off and prop them up against the stove to dry... socks too."

It was an unusual way to be greeted by a patient, but I needed to get those frozen boots off if I wanted to keep my toes. Ben took my wet socks and draped them across the stove. There was a hiss as Ben flipped them back and forth like he was frying an egg and soon the odor of cooking wool filled the room. I hoped he wouldn't order me to take off my wool slacks, even though they were soaking wet.

At first glance, Ben looked content and comfortable. A full head of thick white hair matched his full beard. His ruddy cheeks made his smile bright. His sky blue eyes twinkled when he spoke. "I didn't expect you to come out in this here storm, Kate," he said. "You know me better than that," I replied. "A little bit of snow wouldn't keep me from seeing you."

Once my hands were warm enough, I removed his dressing to reveal a bright pink, nicely healing surgical site. The incision line was a long one, starting at his breastbone and extending halfway around his back. I cleaned the site with an antiseptic, applied antibiotic ointment and covered it with a fresh, sterile dressing. With my stethoscope, I listened to his clear breathing while in my bare feet; a first in nursing care for sure, I thought to myself with a smile. I counted his antibiotics and pain medicines, and refilled the bottles from my stock supply.

"How are you feeling, Ben?" I asked.

"Fine, darling," replied Ben, "Bo and me, we are doing just fine."

Ben's prognosis wasn't good. The cancer had spread into his lymph nodes and bones. His time was limited and he knew it, but he was at peace with his condition. "Just gonna wait it out," he had told me before. "The old man with the sickle is gonna have to come fetch me, I ain't gonna go looking for him."

"Are the pills keeping the pain at bay?"

"Oh, now don't you go fretting about me and pain," he said. "At my age, everything is gonna give you a pain every now and then. I figure there are people a lot worse off than me. Look at the poor children starving. Their bellies pain them more than this cancer will ever pain me."

"Ben," I said, "I want you to tell me if the pain medicines stop working, OK?" I knew they would not help as his cancer spread over time. "I tell you everything, Kate," he answered. "You know more about me than Bo. I just thank the good Lord for your help." I felt a tug at my heartstrings. I had grown fond of this old man and was pained that he did not have long to live.

"It's a privilege to help you, Ben," I told him. "I want you to drink more liquids and keep a pail of water close to the stove to put some moisture into the dry air. It will help you breathe easier. And if you want anything, just ask."

He took my hand, brought it to his bearded cheek. "Can you sit a spell before you gotta go back out there in that storm?"

I looked out the frosted window. It was still daylight, but the storm was not letting up. I told him, "I can stay for a while, Ben, but I need to leave before the roads become invisible."

"Why shucks gal," he said jovially, "you can stay up here with me and Bo. Bo will keep you real warm." My stomach did a flip flop just thinking about Bo snuggling up to me. I was glad Ben couldn't read my thoughts. "Thanks Ben," I said, "but I need to be in town in case other patients need me."

Ben challenged me to a game of checkers, which turned into three, and he beat me each time with no effort. "Ben, you trounced me," I told him. Laughing he said, "Well I reckon I can unless the cancer gets to my brain." He glanced out the window. "Wow, look at that pure white snow piling up against the house. Like God's ice cream. Sometimes when the winds come a-howling, the snow drifts up against the doors and I can't get out."

I asked him how he spent his days and nights alone with the cold winds howling around the cracks in the doors and windows, buried in the snow.

"Most days I sit here in my rocking chair and look out the winders and watch the wild life go by. Deer roam on my little piece of land. Look out there right now, you see that doe?" I saw the beautiful animal standing close to the side of his house, looking like a picture from a greeting card. Ben joked, "I'd invite her in, but Bo doesn't like it when I look at another animal. Reckon he's jealous?" I smiled and he went on. "I never have been lonely up here. Got Bo, food to eat, things to read. What else would I want?"

Finally, I told Ben that if I wanted to make it down the mountain, it was now or never. He handed me my scorched thermal socks. They were dry and stiff. As I sat down on the edge of his bed and slipped on my socks and boots, I took another look around the rooms to see if he could use anything else to help make his days and nights more comfortable. I felt a sudden pang of pain as I realized that I would probably be the one to find him when his time came. But he had told me more than once that he wasn't afraid of death. He spoke of it as the inevitability it was that would claim us all at some point. "Ain't nothing to be scared of," he would say. "When you are dead you are dead."

Ready to go, I gave Ben a hug, Bo a pat on his shaggy head and opened the door to a whiteout. It took forty-five minutes of hard work to get back to my car. The roads were covered, icy and almost impassable. On the road, I had to stop to put chains on my tires. The ice caused my windshield wipers to freeze, and again I had to ride with the window down. The usual one-and-a-half hour drive home took four hours. I was never so happy to see my house. I dragged myself inside, peeled off the many layers of soggy clothes, and got into a hot shower. Happiness filled my tired, chilled body.

I slept well that night. As I gave in to sleep, I had a picture of Ben and Bo cuddled together in their warm house sleeping safely and comfortably and tried to figure out which of us gave the other more courage to face another day and the rest of our lives, and I smiled as I drifted off to sleep. Yes, I slept well that night in my comfortable home. And I was sure that Ben, old, in pain and facing death, was sleeping just as well in his.

A resident of Georgia, Kay Cavanaugh is a retired registered nurse educator who has worked in hospitals as well as community, rural, teaching, and home health nursing.

Lessons Learned

Tom Brown

"The tumor is malignant." Those four words changed my life forever. The tumor was in the right breast of my wife, Barbara. She had inflammatory breast cancer, one of the rarest and most aggressive varieties. After the initial consultation with Barbara's oncologist, she and I sat down and developed a strategy of how we were going to deal with her disease. It was a simple plan: Barbara would be the patient and I would be the caregiver. We vowed to fight the disease and beat breast cancer.

I took our plan very seriously and followed it to the letter. As the caregiver, I did some things right and some things wrong. One right thing I did was to keep copious notes in a daily journal. I wrote down every detail of her treatment, including the type and amount of drugs that she took and the date and time she took them. I noted how she was feeling and documented any physical change, such as a spike in temperature, loss of appetite, nausea, pain or discomfort. There were several times during her treatment that the doctors needed the exact information I had in my journal. I would never have remembered all of it if I hadn't written it down.

Unfortunately, Barbara lost her battle in August of 1994, twenty-one months after her diagnosis. But we did all in our power to beat it. And I learned that being a caregiver means developing the ability to juggle many things every day. Yes, it was hard work, but it was worth it every step of the way. Here are a few of the most important lessons I learned.

Communication. This is probably the most important job and perhaps the most difficult to accomplish by the caregiver, particularly if the caregiver is a man. After diagnosis, the cancer patient will have to live with the physical, emotional and social consequences of having cancer. The caregiver must be able to listen to the needs of the patient effectively. Listen to her fears and be supportive. There are no magic answers. Be mindful that men and women generally communicate differently. Women often express their feelings more openly. When your loved one is talking, listen intently before offering a response. Sometimes she only wants you to hear how she feels and is asking for support, not advice. A simple hug and telling her "I understand, and will always be here for you," is all the response that is needed. She still needs to hear that you love her and always will.

Be mindful of the relationship you have developed with your loved one. If you were not good communicators before the cancer, don't expect to become great ones overnight; it might take some time. But both of you must make an effort to express your feelings. If you were good communicators, build on that relationship. This period in your life will be one of the most stressful you will ever endure, and the ability to understand each other is essential in order to get through it.

Finally, remember that there are other family members who must be included in what is happening. If there are children at home, keep them in the loop. Parents, siblings and friends are important too. They will want to know how the both of you are doing.

Be prepared for the pitfalls. There will be hurt feelings. You or the patient will say something that will be taken the wrong way. As the caregiver, you will try your best to give support and make sure the patient is comfortable. But you will be tired and stressed. The patient can mistake your tone of voice and be hurt by what you say. The patient too will be under constant stress. There will be times when she just does not know what to say. Tell her that it is okay. Offer up an alternative to talking about her feelings, such as writing them down in a daily journal.

Educate yourself. Most male caregivers have no idea what is involved in caring for a loved one who has breast cancer. It is imperative that the caregiver learn as much about the disease as possible as quickly as possible. There are hundreds of sites on the Internet devoted to the subject. The cancer treatment facility that you are using has useful brochures and pamphlets to help you better understand breast cancer.

You should learn as much as you can about the treatment your loved one will undergo. I suggest taking a tape recorder to every meeting with your doctors and ask for their permission to record the session. At the very least, you should keep your own journal with very detailed notes including the date, time, type and amount of drugs that your loved one is taking. There is a very good chance that she could develop an infection and have to be hospitalized. With your notes you can easily tell the attending physician what medication she has taken and when. You will have to be the one to educate the rest of your family and pass along the important information on your loved one's treatment. Try not to shield your loved one from your family and friends. Knowledge is power. The more that select family members know about the disease and treatment, the more they will be able to rally the kind of support that is needed. They will be able to anticipate when extra help or a meal or a visit is most needed.

Take care of yourself. Regardless of your age and physical condition, as a caregiver you will experience both emotional and physical stress. You will feel shock, anger, fear, sorrow, guilt and maybe even hate, just to name a few. If you are a full-time employee, you will have to balance your work with taking care of your loved one. There are domestic responsibilities of tending the house, cooking, etc. If there are children at home, they need your attention also. Caregiving is demanding and stressful regardless of what the circumstances are. Your journal, which can be as simple as a spiral notebook, isn't just a good place to keep track of the details of your loved one's treatment, but your own emotions as well. Take some time at the end of each day and jot down your feelings. It is a way of venting, and it is useful. And you must take care of your physical health. If you are not eating or sleeping properly, it will eventually affect your judgment and your health. If you get a cold or the flu and cannot care for your loved one, seek help from a family member or a friend. This backup caregiver should be involved from the beginning so they can step in at a moment's notice to make the transition. It would also be very helpful to find a friend or family member to look out for your well-being. Ask them to check on you daily, even if it is just a phone call to see how you are doing. You need it and deserve it.

Come to grips with reality. I have been a problem solver my entire life. I am not always successful and I make mistakes on occasion. But I enjoy a hard challenge and take great pleasure when I complete a task. The challenge of helping my wife beat cancer was a problem I never thought I would have to face. It just always seemed that since we were such a happily married couple, we would enjoy the golden years together. I had a very difficult time knowing that I couldn't do a thing to cure Barbara. All I could do was fight along with her and provide as much comfort and support as I could. During our journey, I did a lot of soul searching and philosophical pondering about the meaning of life in general. I found that I had a very hard time focusing on anything but the battle with cancer. It was all-consuming.

But I also found that I had strengths I didn't know I had. When you are at the lowest ebb in your life, somehow you can find the strength to carry on. I found that I was much more pleasant with people than I ever had been before. At the same time, I found myself wishing that someone else had my problems. I would see couples in perfect health and ask, "Why not them?" Not that I actually wanted them to have cancer, but I just wanted it taken away from us. I guess I was just really angry and bitter that others had the perfect life and ours had been shattered.

Keep a positive attitude. This is easier said than done, but vital to the role of a caregiver. There are going to be those days when your loved one is so sick she can't get out of bed. There might be times when her white blood count drops too low and infection sets in. Your loved one will probably lose her hair and gain a lot of weight. Depending on the treatment your doctor recommends, there could be an operation to remove a part of or the entire breast. You may find during the treatment that the cancer has spread to another part of her body. Depending on your financial situation, you may find that money is a very big factor in making decisions about treatment. There are many other things that will occur that will bring you down and keep you from that positive attitude.

During our time of fear, anger, bitterness, sorrow, depression and hatred of what we had been dealt, I never gave up hope. One look at my beautiful wife was all that I needed to keep me going strong and hoping for the best. Barbara's spirit and character gave me strength and courage. She faced the cancer with complete confidence that one day, it would all be over and we could get back to the happy routine that we both cherished so much. Granted, it would be a different life, because we would always live with the fear that the cancer would come back. But we vowed to each other that we would take it one step at a time. And the saddest part of it all was that we had very few choices except to do exactly what we were doing at the time. There was no magic cure.

All of this and more falls directly on the shoulders of the caregiver. Will it stress you out? Of course it will. But keep in mind that the crisis can be dealt with efficiently. Keeping the patient comfortable, informed and getting the best care you can provide are of paramount importance. Everything else takes second place. Keep in mind at all times that breast cancer, no matter what type, is a very dangerous and deadly disease. When you feel overwhelmed, reach inside of yourself for strength or call that friend whose job is to look out for you. If you practice a religious faith, relying on your beliefs can help.

Don't expect to be perfect. You will make mistakes along the way. But learn from your mistakes, and improve. Don't dwell on them too long. Make adjustments to your plan and move forward. It takes time to learn how to be a successful caregiver. Believe me, your loved one will appreciate every little thing you do for her.

And the simplest thing—but one of the most important—is to simply say, "I love you."

Thomas Brown is the author of *Men Bleed Too: A Compelling Story About One Man's Struggle to Help His Wife Fight Breast Cancer*, which chronicles his role as caregiver to his wife Barbara. His follow-up book, *She Taught Me to Laugh Again*, details life beyond the grieving.

I Didn't Get the Memo

Karen Laven

No one ever sent me the memo about what to do when you are squeezed in next to your mother in a tiny, pungent doctor's office, waiting to hear why there happened to be a shadow on her X-ray and a liter of fluid in her lungs. There was no note that told me what to say after her longtime physician popped in and informed my sixty-nine-year-old mom that the reason for all her complications was that she had lung cancer, complete with a hefty, inoperable tumor inside the left lobe.

The long-haired, blonde, blue-eyed doctor informed us that even though Mom had quit smoking ten years ago, she now had a specific mumbo-jumbo type of cancer that looked to be Stage IV.

Huh?

I recall asking the woman in white before us what the hell Stage IV meant. She hesitated. I piped in, "Wouldn't Stage I be the worst?" No? Oh. Nevertheless, isn't there a Stage V for those who are really bad?

We were told that Stage IV covers that dire scenario just fine. I don't remember what I said after that, but I do remember feeling remarkably distant and nauseated. I remember the beauty queen with a stethoscope prescribing Ativan for Mom and handing me a referral for a cancer specialist. What was the point in seeing a specialist if there wasn't anything that could be done? I wanted to ask, but I didn't. I recall wanting to ask the doctor if her mom was alive and well.

That maddeningly sunny September afternoon, as I drove home the person who had raised me, I kept thinking that this wasn't fair—for me. I'd already lost a parent, and right now I desperately wanted my dad. No such luck: he'd died of a heart attack fifteen years earlier.

"I miss your father," Mom said, tears spilling over. I couldn't reply; my throat closed. "I'm so lucky I have you," she added with a smile.

Lucky to have me? The person who has somehow found a way to feel sorry for herself at your terminal diagnosis?

That was the beginning of many thoughts and feelings that would humble and sadden me. Mom was smiling. I couldn't smile. I could barely drive. How could she smile? She not only could, she smiled every day throughout the next fourteen months.

I, however, undertook the drama side of it all. When I was apart from Mom, I'm ashamed to say I often cried, screamed and wailed at the unfairness of my life. I had friends and relatives who not only still had their moms around—in great health—but their fathers too. Why did they get to have both their parents while I would soon have neither?

How atrocious was I? Was I secretly wishing that they would lose a parent? Would that make my loss easier? Would that make everything "fair"? My Lord, what was my mother's cancer diagnosis doing to me?

The compassion within me slipped into high gear to help my mother prolong and enjoy what was left of her life. But I was completely spent when out of her sight. I cringe at my selfishness throughout much of Mom's cancer experience. While helping her keep up with shopping and cleaning and took her to her doctor appointments and chemo treatments, I became enraged at my siblings for not pitching in more. I used guilt tactics—whatever I could—to reach them. I wanted someone to help me help Mom. I wanted them to worry about her, wipe her face after she vomited and get angry like I did when she would let herself suffer by not taking her pain pills.

Now that I look back, I think my siblings were afraid to tip the boat. After all, I had everything under control, right? I became very knowledgeable about Mom's treatment and what she needed as far as pills and other cancer-related issues. Believe me, I let my brother and sisters know it.

The truth is, Mom and I had always been close. We did most of our grocery and clothes shopping together. We held word game tournaments. We baked cookies. But I hated when she'd meander into a shoe store—which was a given if there was one within sight. She'd pick up a sandal, a pump and a boot and then ask the salesman if they all came in narrow and I'd stand behind her, tapping my foot impatiently. She also had a way of cajoling me into playing Scrabble with her when I should have been working on my feature story for the paper, and rubbing it in when she won.

As the months edged by, the shopping sessions decreased and then stopped altogether. I was out alone now, picking up her necessities and passing right by the shoe store. Then came the time she could only make it out of the house to go to church... and then not even for that. It was at this point when the Scrabble game started collecting dust.

Finally, when she lay in my son's bedroom, atop a hospice bed, the purple tide creeping within her fingers and toes, she continued to fight and moan in pain. She was given more morphine, and she still had more pain. Finally her breathing liquefied and she called for me from down the hall.

I walked in and stood by her side. I'd think that each breath would be her last, but over and over, another breath followed. Minute after minute, she clutched life and the pain that it contained. I was in agony seeing her agony. She hadn't been cognizant for hours. She took another bubbling breath and then another. I didn't know if she could hear or understand me, but I leaned down and whispered into her ear: "Mom, your pain is killing me."

She then did something that must have taken phenomenal strength. She clenched her mouth shut, refusing to take those breaths that a body automatically clings to, even in the throes of death. Before I could realize what I'd done, she was gone. She had gone to save me more agony.

I think that if I had gotten that memo—the one to tell me what to do to help a loved one through their terminal cancer diagnosis—it would have done me good if it had said, Do what's right. Don't ask why others are or aren't doing this, or what's fair. If others want to help you, let them. If they aren't able to, for whatever reason, don't allow this to tarnish your relationship with them or their relationship with the person who has cancer. Be honest about what terminal means. It is excruciating, but don't allow yourself to believe you will have plenty of time later to be a good person. Be as good a person as you can be now. That doesn't mean perfect. It won't happen. Just be your best. That means be there for them.

Yes, you will become agitated and exhausted and frightened, but you will also have the chance to make their days, and what remains of your own life, better. Don't be condescending. Keep humor, compassion and your basic relationship intact. If you don't do this, your conscience will remind you about it over and over until your own time comes to pass.

Shut your mouth and open your heart as you drive them to the shoe store and don't complain about how boring it is and how long they're taking looking for that darn size 7-1/2, narrow loafer.

Above all, play Scrabble every single day and rub it in when you win.

Karen Laven's poetry, articles and essays have appeared in magazines around the country. After seven years writing for a Minnesota newspaper, Karen moved to Kentucky, where she lives with her husband, two sons and their toy poodle.

(continued from page 12)

The History and Rationale of Palliative Care and Hospice

Palliative care is therapy that focuses on decreasing pain and suffering by providing treatments for relief of symptoms, along with comfort and support, for patients of all ages. Palliative medicine was first recognized as a medical specialty in Great Britain in 1987. This discipline grew out of the *hospice care* movement which started in the 1960's and 70's. Hospice care, which involves helping ill individuals and their families during the last period of life, is often a key part of palliative care. Over time, the palliative care model has been extended to apply not only to patients who are clearly at the end of life but also to those with chronic illnesses that, although not imminently fatal, cause significant impairment in function, quality of life, and independence. Palliative care for patients with serious illness is no longer seen as the *alternative* to traditional, life-prolonging care. Instead, it is viewed as part of an integrated approach to medical care.

Palliative care should begin as early as possible when a serious illness is diagnosed, working alongside the primary doctors, whether they be oncologists, heart specialists, pulmonary doctors, geriatricians, neurologists, or any other specialty. Palliative care is not characterized by less care or by withdrawal of care; palliative care is not "giving up." On the contrary, palliative care may involve intensive and highly sophisticated medical interventions, albeit ones intended to relieve suffering or improve quality of life. Hospice is limited to the very end stages of life, as stipulated by Medicare.

Palliative care and hospice share similar philosophies; both are delivered by an interdisciplinary team of healthcare professionals, and both can be delivered in a variety of settings. Palliative care differs from hospice care in that it can be provided at *any time* during an illness, may be combined with curative treatments, and is independent of the third-party payer. Hospice, on the other hand, is stipulated by Medicare to provide care for patients who have a likely survival of six months or less.

Prognosis and Palliative Care

Prognostication, or predicting the length of survival of the chronically ill patient, is more of an art than a science in medicine. For example, a patient dying of colon cancer usually has a long period of stable functional performance, then several months of progressive functional decline and weight loss just before death. In contrast, most heart failure patients experience a lengthy, progressive decline in daily function, with periodic bouts of severe symptoms and disability and multiple hospital admissions for exacerbation and for adjustment of treatment. Death often occurs suddenly, and relatively unpredictably, from *cardiac arrhythmia*, abnormal electrical activity in the heart. In a landmark study of the subject, heart failure patients were given surprisingly long prognoses even up to the day before death: the median prognosis on the day before death was a 50% chance of living two months.

Because it is not possible to consistently and accurately predict the timing of death, palliative care should be incorporated early in a patient's course of illness, even in the face of substantial uncertainty about prognosis. As disease progresses, the goals of care usually change accordingly, with the balance shifting from curative to palliative. Also, because it is difficult to accurately predict when someone has a prognosis of six months or less, referral to hospice tends to happen late or not at all. It is important for physicians to know that they can refer a patient to hospice as long as they think the patient has an *estimated* survival of six months or less. In this way, the patient can benefit from the comprehensive services that hospice provides. If the patient lives longer than six months, the physician is not penalized, the patient and the family are often happy, and whether the patient continues to be terminally ill can always be reassessed.

(continued on page 77)

Always Treasure Today

Michael Steven Edwards

To hear a doctor say you only have a few months to live must sound unbelievable to anyone. It was no different for my father. After a yearly physical followed by some additional tests, his doctors told him he had lung cancer and only six to eighteen months to live. He had been a heavy smoker most of his adult life but had successfully quit ten years before. His doctors told him the cancer was not a direct result of smoking.

I learned about Dad's diagnosis when he unexpectedly came to my office. I usually saw my family only on the major holidays, such as Christmas or Thanksgiving. Even then, I kept my visits as brief as I could manage, always using the excuse that I had some important engagement to keep. The truth was, I couldn't stand the tension I felt being around them, and later on, I couldn't be away from alcohol for more than a few hours without beginning to shake and sweat.

"The results say I might have cancer," he told me that day, "but they're still running tests." I could see the fear in his eyes. A vulnerability that I had never seen in him before stirred my heart. It was more than my usual feelings of overwhelming guilt and rejection. This was something very different. It evoked in me feelings of worry and concern for him that I didn't know I had. I felt a need to be close to him and what I had always assumed had been my anger and hatred towards him began to melt. I did not want him to die with us still at odds and I wanted to make sure he knew that, deep down, I loved him.

I made an effort to spend time doing yard work and other chores at his house on my free days. I had to show him I cared. My drinking was no secret and it disappointed him, but I went out there anyway. He clung to the hope that he would be cured or at least have the disease arrested so he could relax and enjoy all of the things he had saved up for all his life. I learned from this whole experience that you'd better live your life in a reasonably happy way today. The "magic day" you wait for, to let yourself loose to enjoy all of those things for which you worked so long, may never come.

Dad ended up living for just over four years from the day he told me of his diagnosis, and he was able to see many remarkable things. I think the proudest day of his life was the day of my sister's wedding. It was a huge affair and he didn't nickel and dime it. I was asked to usher at the wedding two months before, a gesture that utterly broke my heart. The wedding was to take place in Santa Fe, New Mexico. It was to be a week-long event with rehearsals and dinners and entertaining, with lots of people to meet. This meant I would be out of my element and not in control of my time, an alcoholic's worst nightmare.

My alcoholism had progressed to daily drinking. It was a seven-day-a-week physical addiction over which I had no control and of which I was terribly ashamed. There was no way I could participate in the rehearsals and meet everyone without somehow embarrassing my family. Little did I know that a huge change in my life, by which God would enable me to get sober, would happen within weeks. It happened, and I have remained sober ever since. God works in ways that are indeed mysterious, marvelous and magnificent. I was able to be the most awkward, nervous usher you have ever seen, but I was so glad to be a part of it all.

The wedding was beautiful. Dad was asked to make a speech at the reception. He was extremely nervous. Of course he left his notes at the hotel. The truth is, he had given speeches and talks in front of some of the most powerful executives and government officials in the country. But this was the one that mattered. I told him funny stories and got him laughing and he pulled it off beautifully.

Dad went through many changes as the cancer spread. He was able to fight it with chemotherapy in the early days. I was so proud of him when he came to the country club for Thanksgiving dinner. He'd lost his hair but he made it. In my opinion, that would be difficult for anyone, but especially for someone as self-conscious as Dad.

Later, the cancer spread to his brain and he began radiation treatment. Compared to a year of chemotherapy, the side effects from these treatments were less severe. Still, his breathing was worsening, and we had to be very careful to shield him from any type of infection. He needed oxygen when he was at home. At times, Dad would have his breathing treatments and then be up and running around, shopping, seeming happy, as if he were perfectly healthy. Other times he was very difficult to deal with and in a terrible mood, or just sick and out of it.

He was hospitalized a few times during his fight with cancer, usually for an infection and once, in the third year, for a heart attack. Then came the day his blood pressure fell to almost nothing. It would not maintain its normal range, and after being rushed by ambulance to the emergency room, he was kept for observation.

I was able to devote most of my time to caring for him. I was at the hospital every night the first week. One night, we had a talk that laid everything on the table. There were no more secrets after that and he told me he was proud of me. When I told him I was proud of him, he asked me why. He never realized how lucky I felt, having such an accomplished dad. He told me he wished he could have done something to have changed or helped me early on. I told him the truth was that I would have turned out the way I did no matter what family raised me. I honestly believe that. Then he changed the subject, so we didn't get too emotional.

His cancer spread to his bones through his bloodstream, and his doctor wanted to do a spinal tap to find out if it had progressed to his spine. The following day, I was with him when he was told the results: he was now beyond the possibility of successful treatment. I saw the look of a condemned man in his eyes. He really hadn't accepted the possibility of death until then. I was glad I was there and that he wasn't alone.

My parents lived in a very exclusive, gated golf course community, and Dad's doctor was a neighbor. Dad tried to make small talk with him about improvements in the neighborhood; I could sense the doctor keeping my dad at arm's length. I felt so sorry for Dad right then. He was trying to have a dignified conversation with one of his peers, all the while feeling unequal because of his prognosis.

I wanted to jump inside him and scream out how damn dignified he should feel for all of the great things he had accomplished! He didn't need to feel bad about dying; he should have felt great about how he had lived his life. But he didn't. He had lost perspective on what mattered and what didn't. It enraged me. He seemed like a little kid just trying to make conversation to ease his fears of the unknown. He was terrified of dying, he was in a situation beyond his control and he knew it. And I knew there was nothing I could do to fix it.

Dad was never a religious person but he did start watching religious services and shows on television at the hospital. I was able to share with him the miracles that had led to and followed my getting sober. I think this had a profound effect on him, or it at least allowed him to see the huge change that had come over me. The same minister who performed my sister's wedding shared something with Dad about the Apostles' Creed that was very significant to him, but only they knew what that was.

Now it was time to rest, but first we had to move him home. He was in intense pain by this time, as the cancer had begun to close his airway. There was no treatment other than radiation, which would keep his airway open only for a few more weeks. But he wanted to go home: my sister would be bringing her new baby home in six days, the day after Christmas. I helped transport him to and from the hospital on the Med Bus each day for radiation though the entire process. It was unbearable for him, and I thought it did more harm than good. But he wanted to make it long enough to see the baby. Throughout all of this, he and I became closer and closer, with him now dependent on me. He died Christmas Day. Although he hadn't lived to see his grandchild, I know that Dad's determination to see him kept him alive a little longer. So in this sadness I try to hold onto the memory of our treasured moments together. Those moments were far too few, but the love we both felt during that time will last forever.

Michael Steven Edwards is a writer from Oklahoma City, Oklahoma. He divides his time between helping people less fortunate than himself and writing, and he tries to live each day as if it was the only one that existed.

Part II
Commitment

...for the caregiver often means "going the distance" as roles change, relationships evolve and unexpected challenges arise.

Strange Silence

Nicole Drumheller Gargus

There are details of that night which have escaped me. But there are others I'll never forget. I woke up to the sound of my husband opening his gun case in our closet. Immediately my stomach started to turn. "Nathan, what are you doing?" I asked. He took his West Point class pistol out to the living room. I remember the strange silence...

I quickly got out of bed and went to see what was happening. It was dark. Nathan was sitting in his computer chair. He had his loaded gun pointed to his head. My heart pounded nearly out of my chest, but my body froze. Our eyes met in the moonlight shining through our half-shaded windows. He said, "I don't want to live like this. I'm not a man anymore." I carefully moved towards him and gently put my hand on his knee. His hand did not budge; his trigger finger was steady as he leaned his head closer to the barrel of his loaded gun. He closed his eyes.

"Sweetheart," I said in a soft, comforting tone, "please...let's talk about this." I felt like I was out of my body in this moment. I was filled with fear and regret. It had been such a long, hard journey since Nathan's injury. We'd grown together through my experience of caring for him...even as it had been tearing him apart.

Tears started streaming down my face. In my mind, I was asking God's forgiveness for all of my shortcomings as a wife. I was begging Christ for the strength to get through this moment. I silently prayed for the wisdom to find the right words to save my husband's life. All of the arguments we had in the past were meaningless now and the last ounce of resentment I was harboring took flight from my soul. If Nathan pulled that trigger, I would lose my soulmate, my life's happiness. How would I go on living without him? Finally, he spoke.

"Please go outside. Let me do this thing. You will be happier and find someone better when I'm gone. You deserve better than me. I do not want to live anymore. I'm done."

I moved my hand from his knee to his face, and as I looked him in the eyes, I said sternly, "You are not done and you are not broken. There is life beyond the Army. You can and will find a new direction." My words must have reached into his aching soul, because for the first time since I met him, he allowed his tears to flow. As my husband wept I leaned into him and kissed his cheek. I longed to take his pain into myself; I would carry the weight of his suffering gladly just to see him smile again. I felt his tears fall on my shoulder. Memories of our life together before his injury flashed through my mind...

I remember the moment he realized he was falling in love with me: it was New Year's Eve 2001 when he said, "Nicole, I've never met a girl who understood me so well." I fell in love with Nathan quickly, but I remember holding that truth inside myself and waiting for him to express those magical words "I love you" first. One day he found the words to tell me he wanted to join the Army Special Forces; he wanted to become a Green Beret. If he was accepted into the Special Forces he would be deployed eight to nine months a year to the most dangerous places anyone can volunteer to go. I shivered at the thought of my sweetheart not only being deployed more than he was home, but his regularly being put in harm's way. Then he asked, "If I go will you wait for me?"

I was angry, sad, and hurting inside. Yet his decision made me love him even more. I realized that I had fallen in love with a man of integrity, a man willing to die for his country, his soldiers, and a man who put others above himself. I knew understanding and unconditional love from me were what he needed most. My life with Nathan was going to be a challenge, but I loved him and I was not willing to walk away. This was a lifetime commitment.

On the fateful day of Nathan's injury, he called me while he was lying on the ground at a civilian drop zone in South Carolina. It was only a week before he and his platoon were scheduled to deploy to Bosnia. His voice was steady. "Baby," he said, "I don't think I will be going to Bosnia." I assumed he had broken his ankle or that some other fairly minor injury had occurred. I was wrong. Nathan had broken his back. His goal of joining the Special Forces, and his Army career, were over.

Nathan was suffering immensely from the pain of a rare severe thoracic spine injury: his spine was literally shattered, and he had a severe concussion. Doctors feared he could possibly be paralyzed. Nathan's Dad called me that night. Fighting back tears, he asked himself out loud, "Who will take care of my son if he is paralyzed?" Without hesitation I answered, "I will, Sir."

In the next few days I was by Nathan's side at the hospital, waiting to talk with him as he came in and out of consciousness. In the months following his injury, Nathan was grateful to be able to walk, and he was also aware of the fact that he was fortunate not to have had debilitating head trauma from his accident. However, he was determined to get back into top physical shape again and still try out for the Special Forces; he was not giving up on his goal no matter who told him it was time to let go of it.

Although I felt the pain of this loss, it was Nathan who suffered most. Nathan's back pain was beyond what most people could tolerate and his fevers from the pain sometimes kept him in bed for over a week at a time. He tried to run again, but the pain he woke up with the next day was indescribable. His dreams were shattered and he fell into the depths of a dark depression. Once, when he was very depressed, he confessed to me, "Nicole, you are my only reason to live." I could not believe what I heard. For so long I had depended on Nathan to be my strength. Before he'd been driven by his deep need to say these words aloud, I'd never realized that I gave his life meaning. It was scary to think that I alone was his hope at this crucial moment. But I felt a wave of strength rise within me. Suddenly *I* was the strong one. To my surprise, the weight of that responsibility didn't frighten me; in fact, it somehow lent me great courage.

Nathan and I were married during this time and I moved to Georgia shortly after our wedding. I dedicated myself to being a housewife and taking care of my husband. But it was draining. We were in and out of hospitals, we spent endless hours at doctor's offices, and we went many months without being able to truly enjoy life. "It's not worth it," a cousin had warned before we got married. "You should not marry an injured man." Those negative words haunted me as I lay awake at night, exhausted, long past giving all I thought I had to give. I would run my fingers through my husband's fine, soft hair, and tears would well up in my eyes. Nathan was the only man I could imagine being married to. He was my true soulmate and my best friend. I expected his depression to pass in time. I never anticipated things to get to the point where my husband would consider taking his own life.

But now here we were, poised in the dark, waiting for him to either pull the trigger—or find the will to keep trying. It seemed like an eternity, the wait in that strange silence. I do not recall exactly what I said to convince him to put his weapon down, but I remember well not being able to breathe in the moments the trigger was halfway pulled.

Finally, *finally*, he slowly moved the gun away from his head. When he at last put it on the floor he took me into his arms and held me for hours. I was so grateful he made the right choice. There in the fading darkness I thanked God for the strength of my own will and the love of this great man in my arms. I reflected on the meaning of our marriage vows and I realized that our love had, and has, the resilience to last. I also realized that by sticking with Nathan through this difficult journey, I had changed. I used to underestimate myself. I had always looked to Nathan as the greater one—not only stronger but more intelligent and above me. I realized these were never ideas Nathan put into my head, but simply my own insecurities and my inner struggle to find self-worth. But I had discovered a bold sense of strength in my heart, and as we lay on the living room floor I promised myself that I would never lose sight of my own person again—and that I would never forget that Nathan found the same strength and love in me that I had found in him.

In the early hours before sunrise, I lay awake with Nathan in my arms. He was sleeping peacefully, and finally I was able to relax there in the welcome quiet of our home. As morning light shone through our windows, I felt a glimmer of hope for us. I knew the beginning of healing was coming for him, and also for me. He would need me to be strong. And I would be—I will be—because he is my husband, and I love him.

Nicole Drumheller Gargus is the wife of a medically retired Army captain. A freelance writer with numerous articles in print and a children's book in the works, she is a graduate of Eastern University and Rosemont College School of Graduate and Professional Studies.

In Sickness and In Health

Mary Potter Kenyon

I dreaded that party. Despite my misgivings and feeble attempts to dissuade her, our oldest daughter, Elizabeth, planned a twenty-fifth anniversary party for my husband, David, and me. I was hard pressed to come up with a valid excuse for not celebrating this impressive milestone. But there was no denying my feelings; I just wasn't that enthused about being a guest of honor. Abby, our youngest at eleven months, was in the midst of teething and more clingy and demanding than usual, and celebrating what felt like a stagnant relationship with David just seemed like another chore on my long to-do list.

My fears were well-founded. The day was a blur for me. Abby hadn't slept well the night before so we were both tired and cranky. Mid-party, Abby started fussing, and nothing I did would comfort her. Finally, exasperated, I strapped her in her backpack and I left my own party. As I walked around the perimeter of the building I contemplated how difficult everything in my life seemed, including my relationship with my spouse. With a flash of irritation and the sense of frustration that had become a constant in my life, I reflected on how I couldn't even enjoy my own party. I continued walking, giving Abby a chance to sleep a little, my thoughts on the anniversary party I'd left behind.

Twenty-five years of marriage to David, eight children, and a continual struggle to make ends meet had taken their toll on us as a couple. I was so busy caring for small children, home schooling, and keeping house, that most mornings I practically shoved David out the door with a perfunctory peck on the cheek so the children and I could begin our real day without him. While I considered this normal for a couple who had been married a long time and had a large family, I couldn't help but wonder if we were missing something, if things could have been different.

When I returned to the party, guests clamored for a photo-op. I slipped the backpack off and handed over the rudely awakened Abby to her older sister, who vainly tried to entertain her while I obliged the request. Abby's renewed crying jarred my already strained nerves. But I played the part of the happy wife well. My face flushed red from my walk in the heat, I pushed back damp tendrils of hair and mugged for the flashing cameras as our guests prompted David and me to feed each other cake. Across the room, Abby screamed for me, and at that moment, I felt as though I were under water, drowning in a sea of discontent.

Later, looking at the photo of David and me, I see my fake smile, eyes like that of a deer caught in the headlights, and wonder why no one else knew how unhappy I'd become, not even David.

Two years later, David was diagnosed with oral cancer. Clutching his hand on the way home from that doctor's appointment, I was struck by how bleak a future without him looked and how terrified I was. At the thought of losing my husband, I realized just how much I still loved him.

It was shocking to see David after the surgery that removed the tumor on his tongue and thirty-two adjacent lymph nodes. The long chain of stitches on his neck made it look as though someone had tried to remove his head. The sight of a breathing tube and the many wires coming out of his neck and body left me reeling. I couldn't stand to see him in pain that first night in the hospital, and with tremendous guilt I rushed home to the children that had been waiting for me all day.

Though I'd never left our children with babysitters before, for eleven straight days I arranged care for them so I could visit David in the hospital. During the seven days he couldn't talk, I learned to watch him for nonverbal clues or waited quietly while he wrote unsteadily on a board propped in front of him. Before all this, I had always waited impatiently for him to finish talking and get to the point. Now I searched his beautiful brown eyes for every little nuance of meaning. I sat by his bed and held his hand for hours. Without the verbal communication, which we evidently hadn't been handling so well in the past few years, I started seeing him in a different light. I saw his strength in handling incredible pain, his gentleness in reaching for my hand, his genuine concern for our children and myself in the questions he wrote.

Once when I arrived for a visit I spotted his writing board on an end table. "*My wife is wonderful*," he'd written in response to a question one of the nurses must have asked. Tears sprang to my eyes. I hadn't been so wonderful in recent years, I thought. During those daily visits in his quiet hospital room, away from the cacophony of our house full of boisterous children, I found myself falling in love with my husband all over again. I spent an inordinate amount of time preparing for our hospital visits, using fragrant lotions on my arms and legs after showering, applying makeup, and dressing in the skirts and tops that I had pushed to the back of my closet in favor of my mom-at-home uniform of loose shirts and leggings. I realized with slight embarrassment that I was courting my own husband.

I became David's caregiver during his recovery from surgery and the six weeks of radiation and chemotherapy treatment, treatments that sometimes seemed worse than the disease. Once he was home from the hospital, I changed the bloody dressings on his wounds, doled out medication, and gave him tube feedings every three hours. Normally squeamish, I found myself doing things I would not have imagined I could do: cleaning David's neck wound with a long cotton swab or wiping away pus that drained from the tube protruding from his abdomen.

In the process of doing these things I began to feel as though it were a great honor and a privilege to care for the person I loved. I found myself reaching out to touch his shoulder as I passed the chair where he sat, taking hold of his hand and kissing his palm, and even kneeling in front of him to rub his feet, something I had never done before. The first time I did this, the surprised look on his face quickly turned to gratified pleasure. It touched me to realize how much he appreciated being cared for, and how little of that care he'd experienced before cancer had entered our lives. I reflected that in all the years he'd brought me my first cup of coffee of the day, I'd rarely done the same for him. When David started chemotherapy, I became his companion every Wednesday for the two-hour sessions, where we held hands and watched television or I wrote while he slept. I looked forward to these quiet times together. The children not only survived being cared for by others, they thrived on the attention paid to them by concerned aunts. More importantly, they watched and learned how much their mother loved their father and how a spouse cares for an ill partner.

My days of caregiving were long and seemed to blend into one another. The combination of chemotherapy and radiation took their toll on David and drained him of energy: it pained me that it was now David handing me the jars to open in our house instead of the other way around. Along with caring for him and the children, everything else seemed to fall on my shoulders. I carted the garbage out, chauffeured David to appointments, cleaned the house, and held the family together through the months of David's cancer treatment. Gradually, David's need for constant care diminished as he regained his strength and recovered. The day he resumed part-time work was a bittersweet moment. As I hugged him goodbye, I could feel how thin his shoulders had become.

It wasn't until he had resumed full-time work and things were on the upswing that I found myself inexplicably falling apart. My nerves were shot. I was anxious and near tears at all times. The kids took the brunt of my moodiness and impatience, with me snapping at them for little or no reason. It was David who noticed my despondency and encouraged me to find a way to take care of myself. I began getting up at 5:00 A.M. every morning for some quiet time for my writing. That helped, but I was still lethargic and irritable. I was amazed when David suggested I try a gym in town. The idea of spending money on something like that seemed decadent. But I joined a local Curves for women and started exercising three times a week. For the first time in my married life, I was learning to take care of myself, and it made all the difference. My anxiety dissipated somewhat and I felt better than I had in years, emotionally and physically.

Early on in our journey through cancer I'd read of survivors who claimed that cancer had been a gift in their lives. I couldn't imagine viewing all that David had to endure as a gift. The invasive surgery? The poisonous chemotherapy? The punishing radiation? A gift? Yet, somehow going through all of the cancer treatment along with my spouse, I feel as though we've been given a second chance. I have never felt closer to my husband nor loved him more than I do now and he says the same of me. I am reluctant to see him leave each morning before work, and I make time for talking with him, or just holding hands. I even bring him cups of coffee in the morning. We are ensured regular dates when I accompany him to doctor's appointments and CT scans, followed by shopping and eating lunch together. We look forward to these times alone together.

Ten months after David's cancer diagnosis and almost three years after she'd thrown our dismal anniversary party, our daughter offered to watch the younger children while her dad and I spent a night alone. For the first time in twenty-seven years, David and I rented a room at a hotel, heralding the beginning of our new life together.

I couldn't have been more excited about this anniversary party for two.

––––––––––––––

Mary Potter Kenyon graduated from the University of Northern Iowa with a Bachelor of Arts degree in psychology. Her writing has appeared in magazines including *Home Education, Backwoods Home, Our Iowa, Woman's World,* and in the book, *Chicken Soup for the Mother's Soul.* Her book, *Homeschooling From Scratch,* was published in 1996. Mary is currently working on a book about the journey through cancer as a couple.

Do You Have Any Brothers or Sisters?

Whitney Sheppard

A few years ago, I hated being introduced to new people because of the inevitable small talk. For example: picture me at twenty-two at a nice local bar where I'm hanging out after work with some friends. A guy buys me a drink and I feel obligated to have a conversation with him. It's light and easy at first, and everything is going well until he asks:

"So, do you have any brothers or sisters?"

I could lie and say no. I could say that I have an older brother and stop right there. At this, I might receive an expectant smile. The guy waits for me to tell him where my brother goes to school, or what he does for a living. When I don't, he assumes that I don't want to talk about him, and from that he assumes that there's been a falling out, and that my brother is somehow estranged from the family.

Which leaves me with option three:

"Yes, an older brother. He's severely autistic. Retarded as well. It's no big deal. I mean, sometimes he has seizures, so I've got to watch his medication pretty closely. My parents are taking care of him now, but I'm going to inherit him down the line, so it's sort of like I'm really the big sister, even though I'm not. Or like I've got a kid. Funny, right? Anyway, it's really no big deal."

It really *is*, and always has been, a big deal.

My older brother Matthew has four years on me, but I have nearly twenty-three years of development on him. Whenever I gently press a hand to Matthew's arm, he flinches and turns away. The resulting groan is annoyed and reprimanding. I can tickle Matthew's sides and carefully slide my fingers through his hair, but he always shudders and glares at me in aggravation. No matter how tender my touch or tentative the connection, my brother pulls away from me.

Matthew has never enjoyed being touched or getting hugs. Touch of any kind is an annoying distraction from eating the carpet or curling into an autistic and antisocial ball. Occasionally, I'll force him into a hug, and if he continues to resist, I take the nearest pillow and harass him with it until he laughs so hard that tears stream down his cheeks. It is how our sibling interaction has always been: fast and prickly and painful, like a smile that's been on your face too long or the headache that accompanies a particularly violent crying fit.

I cut up his food for him, I hold his hand if we're walking outside together, and I change his diapers. If people stare at him, I smile, hold out my hand, and say hello so that they have to notice me and not him. I do understand why people stare. Matthew makes loud noises, and tends to walk by putting all his weight from his left foot to his right, swaying from side to side as he lopes down the sidewalk. He groans. He picks his nose. Some of the faces he makes are so grotesquely unusual that they're unfit for public display. I make those faces right back at him in front of whoever happens to be watching, because Matthew is a perfectly normal planet in my universe. People are allowed to stare, but only for a moment, and if anyone tries to take a gander longer than necessary, they're going to be met with the full force of my teeth showing through my perfect smile.

I've taken care of Matthew for as long as I can remember. Mom and Dad took the brunt of the responsibility when I was younger, but I always had an eye out. While my friends knew that leaving their dolls lying out might result in them being vacuumed or lost, I knew that if I neglected to put dolls away, they would likely be eaten. Many tiny pink shoes, a plastic fireman's helmet, and my favorite coloring book met their end in my brother's voracious mouth, not to mention several pairs of sheets, paychecks, a babysitter's hearing aid, and a rusty nail that caused my mother endless worry the entire time that it was being digested.

When I was little, I took care of Matthew because it meant taking care of myself. I didn't want him to eat my toys any more than I wanted the blame when Mom found Barbie heads in Matthew's mouth. It was just the way things were: not abnormal in the least, I thought. At least not until I started going to school and encountered how small children can be about people who are different from themselves. In second grade, all it took was a few references to "stupid retards" and suddenly the tooth fairy was visiting Timmy Greene a little early that year, and I had earned myself my first and only naughty point of the school year.

"Wow, it must be hard."

You'd think that with all the things that I have to deal with, that particular phrase would be the least of my problems. It never fails to make me bristle. In retaliation I'm torn between particularly poisonous sarcasm and full-out attack. I know that it's not fair of me to throw someone's attempt at pity and empathy back in their face, but my instinct comes out every time. I've gotten good at smiling, saying something along the lines of "Yes, yes it is" and changing the subject, because yes, it is hard.

It's also life. When I was born, I already had Matthew's imperfect puzzle piece in my life. He has always been here, and I can't imagine life without him. It's hardest if I compare myself to friends who have older brothers who speak, wash themselves, and play practical jokes on their annoyed little sisters.

I left my home in the hills of Alabama for an education in Virginia. For nearly a week after I left, Matthew would walk to my room, standing puzzled in the doorway, looking for me. It was then that I knew that I wasn't just a decoration in the family tree of which he was only vaguely aware. I was his sister, and he knew where I was supposed to be. Now, whenever I come home to visit, it takes him about two hours to understand who I am, but once he starts laughing, it's a gleeful, loud, and relieved sound that fills the house. I laugh right alongside him and feed him chocolate that I've brought back for him, whole bars of it that ruin his supper.

I received my Letter of Guardianship in the mail the other day. It means that I'll be taking care of Matthew in the future, after Mom and Dad are gone. I have a piece of paper guaranteeing that he is mine and I am his. I should put the paper in my drawer with other important documents, but it's resting on my desk next to the keyboard and I keep sneaking looks at it.

And you know, I think I'm ready for it at last. Five years ago, I wasn't. Even two years ago, I wasn't, but I've accepted what it will mean for the two of us. I used to think that caregiving was about taking care of Matthew and making sure that he was as healthy and happy as his situation would allow. It meant keeping Barbie shoes out of his mouth and giving him his medication on a rigid schedule and putting him to bed at night.

But an examination of the word's actual structure will reveal a subtler definition. "Care" means to provide attention and support for someone who needs it, but it also indicates an emotional connection between the pair that goes beyond mere sustenance. "Giving" deals with both the act of provision as well as the endless well of generosity that is required of the role. There's no passivity in caregiving, and there's not a robotic fulfillment of duty. You can only smile, shut your eyes, and jump off the cliff into whatever is coming, because it will happen regardless of how prepared you are for it.

A few days ago I was in a bar with my friends, and I was talking to a nice guy about my family. He asked me the question that used to send me into a linguistic panic:

"So, do you have any brothers or sisters?"

I smiled and nodded. "Yes, an older one. His name's Matthew. He's autistic, and I take care of him. What about you?"

When I come home every evening, Matthew sits in his chair, rocking back and forth. His fingers are sticky with saliva and are wetting the arms of his chair. His eyes see nothing, certainly not my approach, because they are staring forward, wide and distracted.

Every night I reach forward and give him a hug, burying my head beneath his chin. He flinches, groans irritably, and tries to push me away, hating hugs with the same fervor as always.

I hold on tighter, my face fierce and my fingers digging into his arms, and not the strongest wind in the world is going to make me to let go.

Whitney Diana Sheppard was born in the Alabamian foothills of the Appalachian Mountains in 1983. She graduated with an undergraduate degree in English from the University of Mary Washington in Fredericksburg, Virginia, and a master's degree in advertising and public relations from the University of Alabama in Tuscaloosa. Whitney currently works at Walt Disney World Resort as a communications specialist and is in the process of writing her first novel.

Love Is Never Too Old

Carla Joinson

When I was a very fresh eighteen, I graduated high school and leased an apartment on the strength of a small savings account and a large faith that I would find a job quickly. I soon discovered, however, that I was not needed at the bank, the grocery store, the newspaper, or at either of the two fast food restaurants in town. Finally, I decided to try for a position I had saved as a dead-last option. Several people had assured me that I could always get a job *there*. *There* was a nursing home, and the position was as a nurse's aide.

The moment I walked through the door to fill out an application, I understood why a position would always be available. The heavy institutional smell almost knocked me backward. Men and women shuffled through the halls. They groaned, chattered, and wailed with varying degrees of purpose and passion. I was scared, and almost turned around and walked out. Then I thought of my bare cupboards and meager prospects elsewhere. I took a deep breath, performed the female equivalent of girding my loins, and went up to the front desk. An hour later, I was told I could start the following week. I wasn't sure if I was happy or not, but the administrator had mentioned free lunches.

The next Monday, I stood in the administration area, waiting for the shift leader to tell me what to do. Directly in front of me was a small man restrained in a padded wheelchair. He obviously had some sort of disease or degenerative condition which demanded the restraint, because he jerked and flopped so uncontrollably he would have fallen onto the floor without it. A few people walked around aimlessly, or sat waiting for breakfast. An elderly woman chanted endlessly, "What'll I do, Hon? What'll I do?" Up to this point, my only exposure to the elderly had been grandparents of sound mind and body. Something about these people, though, seemed so different and troubling, and I knew I'd never be comfortable around them.

A thin, frail man caught my eye. He sat at a table and smiled with peculiar intensity. Occasionally, he gave a healthy yell, then smiled with satisfaction. He frightened me with his random chortles and yelps and mindless grinning. Within the hour, I made the unpleasant discovery that he was one of *my* patients.

Hunched and balding, Eddie was retarded and crippled, his birthplace and age unknown. He was so thin I could feel his ribs when I straightened him up in his chair. I fed him breakfast, but cringed whenever he leaned toward me to follow the spoon. He couldn't speak. By now I had categorized his smiles as leers, his shouts as ravings, and his helplessness as a burden that would bring me nothing but trouble. My only motivation to stick with the job lay in an empty bank account and the knowledge that I could outrun any of my patients.

But like so many other times since then, the Lord was preparing a lesson for me. As time passed, I learned that each patient, or resident as we were told to call them, had a unique personality. Eddie did too. He was the most docile of my residents, and I finally began to appreciate him just for that: I struggled daily with women who thought they needed to go home to tend to their children; men who thought they were in prison; and an assortment of dismayed residents who just didn't know what was going on.

Eddie soon became my patient of choice, although I still got frustrated with him. For one thing, he couldn't tell me when he had to go to the bathroom. I spent half my day trying to anticipate him, and the other half mopping up my mistakes. To be fair, though, I was learning about cleaning up puddles from a lot of people. The difference was that Eddie laughed all the way through the task, instead of swatting at me or running.

I learned that he was gentle beneath the shouts and yelps. He began to smile at me when he saw me each morning, and I was flattered that he recognized me despite his profound impairment. I'd catch his eye sometimes as I whizzed by during my chores, and he'd rock with excitement. In turn, I started kissing the top of his head whenever I had an extra minute. Somehow, he'd gotten a lot cuter.

One afternoon, I had to give Eddie his weekly shave. This task usually fell to the second shift, but they must have had to skip Eddie that week; he looked sad and neglected, and I couldn't bear it. I walked Eddie to a chair in a little waiting room and plugged in the electric shaver. He immediately began screaming. "Eddie," I said soothingly, bringing the buzzing shaver closer. "It's all right, little buddy." Eddie began bouncing in his chair, shrieking and batting at the shaver. Two other aides walked in the room and chuckled at my dilemma.

"He's afraid of the noise it makes," they told me. "You're going to have to use a razor."

Sighing, I switched gears and got a pan of warm water. I lathered Eddie's face while he laughed up at me, and I couldn't help laughing back. But when I brought the safety razor to his cheek, he began twitching frantically.

Ten minutes later, with the help of the other aides, I had Eddie restrained and re-lathered. He was still twitching and shuddering, so I finally tucked his head in the crook of my arm, smashing one side of his face against my waist. He frowned with all his might, but I shaved him anyway. Then I switched sides and got the other cheek, while he yelped and struggled without end. When I was finished, we were both exhausted and streaked with blood from a few minor cuts.

I washed his face and took off his hand restraints, cringing slightly in anticipation of the blow I expected. Free at last, he turned his face to me. He scrunched his lips into a familiar grin, and began chuckling as if we had both been party to a good joke. I was forgiven.

A year passed. Eddie rocked and smiled whenever he saw me coming, and followed me with his eyes whenever I was in the room. The day I left for another job, I was ashamed to think I had once been afraid of him. He gave me my first smile of the morning, and my last one of the afternoon. He never cared if I was in a bad mood, or tired, or preoccupied. And though I only gave him the simplest of physical care, he taught me a lesson I carry to this day. I learned about compassion for the elderly, understanding for the handicapped, and love for people who were different from me. The simple little man who grinned and chuckled so trustingly, gave me perhaps the most unselfish love of my adult life.

He never even knew my name.

Carla Joinson is a freelance writer in Virginia who covers a number of topics for magazines and private clients. She considers her first job in a nursing home to be one of the most important she ever held.

Behind Lace Curtains
Kali J. Van Baale

I sit before a pile of his denim overalls and white underwear, labeling the tags with his initials in black marker like I did for my children when they started school. Two small boxes containing family photos, hygiene items, and a faded crocheted afghan I made decades ago are next to the door, ready to be loaded. Two boxes are all he is allowed to take. I move a sack of his shoes as he stumbles into the room; slippers on the wrong feet even though I taped a large L and R on the top of each one, and I see that the fly of his overalls is open.

"Here, let me help you," I offer, tugging at the metal zipper.

"I love you," he repeats over and over.

"Yes, yes," I say, ever conscious of the time. "We've lost your glasses. Where did you put your glasses?"

Another search begins—under furniture, in closets, on top of cabinets. I check my watch and rub my swollen fingertips which protrude from the end of a dirty white cast on my wrist. During my search, I find that his T-shirt is in the toilet, the remote control is in the microwave oven, and he has poured his morning coffee into the sugar bowl. But no glasses.

"You're sore at me," he says.

"No. I'm not."

"You were sore at me yesterday."

"Yes, yesterday."

"I wet my pants."

"Yes, yesterday."

"I love you," he repeats. "I love you."

"Yes, yes, we're in a hurry." I softly shoo him away. "Now where are your glasses? We can't leave without your glasses."

He sags into his vinyl recliner with a whoosh of air under his weight and dozes off. His favorite recliner, I think—too big for his new room.

There is a pinch between my shoulder blades as I move the kitchen chairs back to the table out of the corner where he has pushed them. I am tired, but there is more to be done. I go to the window and press my forehead to the chilled pane, watch a cardinal eat from my birdfeeder in the backyard. I am wasting time, I know, but cannot help myself. I miss my garden, now overgrown and choked with foxtail and creeping Charlie, the corn patch ravaged by raccoons. I can't deny that my kitchen is also a mess. I see the piles of dirty pots and pans and know that the air in the room is stale. I don't notice so much anymore, but my children have made comments. Our dishwasher has not been fixed since his fall and it is difficult for me to wash the dishes by hand, which I explained to them, to no avail. These days, I am always falling behind. I keep reminding myself of this as I pack his boxes.

"He didn't push me," I had assured my son. "I was trying to catch him. He lost his balance is all. My fault really."

Ridiculous notion, I know, for a woman my age to think she could catch a grown man. Look at the result—both tumbling on top of the opened dishwasher door and me breaking my wrist instead of breaking our fall. There we lay, nearly six hours before my grandson found us, a jumbled pile of old bones on the floor.

"It's too dangerous," my son told me at the hospital. "You can't do this by yourself anymore. We'll get him the care he needs. You can visit any day of the week."

"Yes, yes, I know," I said. And I do know. His disease, his frightening journey of forgetfulness, cannot be helped by my poor eyesight, my bad heart, my brittle bones or paper-thin skin. Even though I know, still...

I pull the long drapes aside and there they are, his glasses, resting neatly on the sill behind the lace curtains. I unfold the earpieces and wipe the smudged lenses on the bottom of my shirt. I gently place them back on his weathered face, now passive with sleep, and smooth down a few long, wispy white strands of his hair with the palm of my hand. He needs a trim. I've always given him his haircuts. I did it in our early years because we never had the money to pay a barber, then later, because he just liked for me to do it. It suddenly occurs to me that I could still do that for him—give him his regular haircuts. When I visit in a few days, I could bring my hair scissors and electric trimmer. He will sit still for me, always calmed by my touch. Yes, I can still do that for him. I am hopeful to think that perhaps there are moments left to be shared between us, no matter where, or how small, or seemingly inconsequential, that I can look towards and wrap my hands about to protect and keep warm.

But for now, I've wasted time again and our time is almost out. I wipe my eyes and return to the stack of clothing, to the boxes where I carefully printed his name on the side, the name I have shared for over sixty years. I hurry to finish before my son arrives to pick us up.

Kali J. Van Baale grew up on a dairy farm in rural Iowa. She is an alumnus of Upper Iowa University and lives outside Des Moines with her husband and two children. She is the recipient of the 2005 Fred Bonnie Memorial Award for Best First Novel for her work of fiction, *The Space Between*.

(continued from page 42)

Settings for the Delivery of Palliative Care

Palliative care may be delivered in a variety of settings, including a hospital, nursing home, hospice, or private home. In some cases, the level of care required will dictate the choice of setting.

Hospitals

Increasing numbers of hospital-based palliative care programs have been developed in recent years to meet the needs of people who are chronically and critically ill and who eventually die in hospitals. A national Center to Advance Palliative Care has been created to provide technical support and resources for hospitals that want to establish such programs. As of 2007, 1,299 hospitals (31%) nationwide provide palliative care programs. This is compared to just 632 programs in 2000. Furthermore, 77% of hospitals with over 250 beds (large-size hospitals) have such a program.

Home Hospice

Hospice is one way to deliver palliative care. Hospice became an official Medicare benefit in 1982 and has grown ever since. From 1984 to January 2008, the total number of hospices participating in Medicare rose from 31 to 3,257, a more than 105-fold increase. Hospice care traditionally has been characterized as "low tech, high touch." But with advances in medical technology and an increasing number of sicker patients, hospice is admitting and caring for more and more patients with complex medical needs. Hospice provides comprehensive services including home nursing, support for the family, spiritual counseling, pain and symptom management, social work intervention, medications for the illness that prompted the referral, medical visits at home, and inpatient hospice care when appropriate. The National Hospice and Palliative Care Organization (NHPCO) estimates that in the United States, hospices admitted over 964,000 patients in 2006 (compared with approximately 340,000 persons in 1994) and that, in 2006, one in three persons who died of all causes were receiving hospice care at the time of death. But it is important for people to know that the vast majority (about 95%) of hospice care is delivered at home. Some people, and many physicians, think of hospice as "going to a place" and therefore do not consider it. For terminally ill people who want to be at home with their loved ones, hospice provides the most direct way of reaching that goal.

Inpatient Hospice
If the patient becomes too ill or their symptoms too difficult to control at home, *inpatient hospice* can be an option. Most hospice programs provide inpatient hospice within a hospital, a nursing home, or a free-standing facility, offering intensive pain and symptom management that is not possible at home.

Nursing Homes
Palliative care can be provided in nursing homes, and increasing numbers of nursing homes strive to do so. Policies governing the coordination of palliative care in nursing homes vary according to reimbursement venues and the availability of trained staff. Many nursing homes coordinate palliative care through local hospices, taking advantage of their skilled hospice nurses and other healthcare professionals.

(continued on page 105)

These Days I Will Remember

Laurie McConnachie

Heartache is watching your father lose his mind in front of you. For the last several years, I have resisted the belief that this was really happening. The harsh truth has finally cornered me, however, and I can't deny the signs any longer. I am trying to get used to saying the full version of what I have been referring to as the "A" word. I speak it with the hesitation of a child learning to enunciate a new sound and trying to comprehend how it applies to his reality. It's not because I don't know how to pronounce it, but because I'm afraid to give it audible validation. The word is Alzheimer's, and it has overturned my world.

My weary feet now follow their own footprints back into the netherworld of neurology, where I spent two years watching a brain tumor eat away at the person who was my mother and where I now see my father's brain also being seized by disease. Focused on my mother's illness, I didn't realize that obscured in its shadow, my father was losing his faculties, too. Alzheimer's is stealing away the connection that we once shared, one that has been a cornerstone of my personal foundation.

Alzheimer's was the last ailment that I thought would affect someone of such intellectual vigor as my father, who skipped two grades in school and went on to do well in university. His sharp mind was one of his most acknowledged attributes. He took on the business and civic worlds with verve, rising to the top of many of the organizations with which he was affiliated.

When I was growing up, every night at dinner my dad would ask my brother and me, "Tell me what you learned today. What is going on in the world?" Later in the evening, he would climb into bed and pick eagerly from a stack of books that perpetually awaited him. Finally, after he read for an hour or two, book resting on his chest and spectacles sliding down his nose, his body would take a break from his inquisitive mind.

The reality of his memory loss hit me when I returned from a long trip to find unpaid bills scattered haphazardly around the house. A man who is an accountant, nationally recognized in his profession and who has never paid a bill late in his life, just doesn't receive notices that his power and phone are about to be shut off. Now I manage my father's finances and his home, arrange for his medical care, and buy his Depends. Now I try to engage the interest of this once sophisticated businessman with ordinary chores such as folding the laundry and unloading the dishwasher.

Sometimes I shake my head and smile when I find a hat in the freezer or a bizarre, yet somehow artful, conglomeration of pebbles, twigs, and grass carefully arranged on my nightstand. Humor, however, cannot always alleviate the ache from finding my father snacking on nuggets of dog food he has scooped up from the bowl or the countless times he has come into my bedroom at three or four in the morning, flipped on the light, wearing mismatched outfits such as a parka over his pajamas, black polished dress shoes with no socks and a golf hat, exclaiming, "Come on, get up! Let's go out for dinner!"

Helping my father to bathe can take all afternoon as I try to convince him that the water won't hurt him. Sometimes he is afraid to get out of the car and will sit in the garage for hours. Then there are the unpredictable times when he is so confused and frightened that he will lash out by yelling, hitting, or biting.

Every night, I take his hand and lead him down the narrow hallway to his bedroom. He insists he is a visitor in this house in which he has lived for more than thirty years. His room is almost bare; most items have been removed due to his obsession with packing everything up and setting it by the front door to take "home." The doors are dead bolted to prevent him from wandering, the keys hidden along with those to the car (a replacement car for the one he drove into a tree three blocks from home and totaled, with no memory of the incident minutes after it happened).

Despite my efforts to ease the way, I feel helpless as I witness my father's constant struggle to maintain his dignity in the face of an illness that is determined to rob him of it. As his memory worsens, my patience must increase exponentially. I repeat and repeat and repeat again. We are no longer able to have a meaningful conversation. In fact, most of our talking together makes little sense; I simply try to follow the train of his tangled thoughts.

Just when I think I'm able to accept the reality of the disease, it will poke at me in new places, testing my willingness and ability to stay the course. Each time, it steals away more of my father, and I must again figure out how to adapt to the latest loss of functioning. My father is with me, and yet I miss him terribly.

Accompanying my newfound courage to say the word Alzheimer's, however, has been the clarity to see that, while my father's mind is failing, his heart is not. His essence remains the same. He still greets people with a smile, handshake, and "How are you today?" He is still the first to open a door or reach for his wallet, even though he no longer carries one. He won't eat his food until he knows that everyone else has some, too. Rarely does he forget to say "please" or "thank you."

I see how gentle he still is when our black Lab, Keira, joins him on the bed at night, filling up some of the space left empty by my mother's death, and together, hand cupping paw, they fall into slumber. Each morning as I pull open the drapes in his room, I hope that again today I will hear him sing and laugh, even if it is a song or joke that only he understands.

Nor has he lost his insatiable curiosity. "Look at that!" he exclaims often on our daily outings, pointing animatedly at a tree, a plane, or even something as mundane as a stop sign. It is as though he is seeing the world for the first time. He is my parent teaching me to see through child's eyes; what was once old is fresh again.

"How did you like the music?" I asked my father recently while driving home from a Celtic concert.

"What music?" he asked blankly.

Sighing into my fatigue, I questioned why I had exerted the effort to get him there if he wasn't even going to remember it. Then a flash in my mind's eye reminded me of the sweetness that seems so inextricably entwined with the sadness of Alzheimer's. I recalled seeing my father merely minutes earlier in the concert hall, whistling and clapping along while tapping his toes to the old Scottish melodies of his childhood. I realized then that he had "been" there and happily so, perhaps even more than I had been.

As I have found myself doing more often lately, I come into the den where my dad spends a lot of his day, sit on the sofa and watch him as he sleeps in the brown leather chair that seems to engulf more of him daily. I take in his presence, never knowing how much longer fate will give me the chance to do so. I breathe in his innocence, and feel the loss of my own that has come from witnessing this man I love dearly slowly fade away before my eyes. I ache for his helplessness, as well as my own that stems from the hard pounding fact that no matter how hard I try, I cannot stop the obliterating trail that Alzheimer's is blazing through his besieged brain. I feel the exhaustion that is deeper than deep and the despair that comes from caring for a man who no longer knows his own name, who talks to his own reflection in the mirror like it is a stranger.

Despite these feelings, however, is the growing awareness that although my father is helpless, his situation is not hopeless. Ironically, the word Alzheimer's, which has daunted me with its implications for years, holds no meaning for the one who bears its affliction. Mercifully, my father is oblivious to his own demise. Forced to live within the confines determined by a disease he does not comprehend, he is still very much alive and, in many respects, one of the most contented people I know. While he has lost most of the skills he once used to navigate through his world, he has developed an uncanny ability, much of the time, to delight in the simple mystery of what remains before him. In those random, fleeting moments when I can push past my own sadness and meet him there, my life is the richer for it.

My father has shared many gems of wisdom with me throughout my lifetime. Perhaps the lessons he is teaching me now as I accompany him on this final journey will prove the most powerful yet. My challenge is to make peace with the pain that is an inescapable part of the end and to embrace the joy that comes from walking by my father's side.

Laurie McConnachie holds a Bachelor of Arts degree and a master's degree in art history and art education from Stanford University and left her career to care for her parents through prolonged and debilitating illnesses. Her writing has helped her find meaning and beauty in seemingly nonsensical suffering and to see the experience from the perspective of the human condition with which we all grapple. Her work has been published locally and nationally. She lives in Seattle with her husband and son. Laurie dedicates this essay to the memory of her parents who taught her to love deeply and live fully, even when it hurts.

For the Love of Rose
Susan Melchione

"*Sangue delle mie vene!*" she called out. The others in the room sat in silence. "*Sangue del mio cuore!*" she called out again. You could hear a pin drop. Rose smiled as she translated the Italian phrases she had just spoken. "'Blood of my veins! Blood of my heart!' This is what my mother said to me as she smothered me with kisses every day."

Rose enjoys sharing her life stories with the other members of the early-stage Alzheimer's group here at the Neuwirth Memory Disorders Program at the Zucker Hillside Hospital Geriatric Center. Many of her long-term memories are joyful. Rose was one of five children born to immigrant parents. They were poor, but no one knew it. Her mother was a dressmaker. For a nickel's worth of material, she said, her mother made her the best dressed girl in school.

One day, while Rose was working with four hundred girls at a brassiere factory, a handsome man asked her where she went for lunch. She had no idea that he was about to become the love of her life. From that day on, Bert sat next to her at lunch and would not leave her side. In 1944, Bert proposed. Rose told her very religious Catholic mother about her engagement to this Jewish man. Without hesitation, her mother asked, "*Tu l'ami?*" which means

"Do you love him?" Rose responded, "Yes, I do!" and her mother took her in her arms and kissed her. Her mother knew that love transcends all.

Bert's love for Rose ran deep. After graduating high school in 1936, Bert had dreams of becoming a veterinarian. He was unable to complete his college education since his parents could not afford the $30 monthly tuition. Bert worked in his father's deli in Brooklyn until his aunt got him a job as a mechanic's helper, also in a brassiere factory. Bert was grateful for the $15 weekly salary. He wanted to learn the trade, but the head mechanic would not teach him. Always believing that there is a solution to any problem, Bert became friendly with the factory foreman, who allowed Bert to stay at night so that he could teach himself about the machines. His diligence paid off. Eventually, they fired the head mechanic and replaced him with Bert.

He also worked hard doing freelance work in the industrial sewing machine business and was proud to support himself and his lovely bride. When his father became ill, his mother suffered a nervous breakdown, and his brother lost his job, Bert supported them all.

Bert and Rose thrived. They had a romantic relationship and they treasured their sons, whom they call their two "jewels." Over the years, Bert developed health problems, including heart problems, emphysema, and prostate cancer. Bert continues to use oxygen at all times and suffers from angina. Rose has suffered for many years with Crohn's disease. Despite this, they manage to enjoy life.

Bert says that he lives by the motto "A bi m'lacht," which is Yiddish for "as long as you can laugh." Bert found it much more difficult to laugh after Rose developed symptoms of Alzheimer's disease in 2002. He could not accept that Rose had an incurable disease. After all, he's the fix-it guy.

Bert had always believed in nontraditional solutions. He subscribed to several alternative medicine journals, all of which agreed that phosphatydylserine (PS), a nutrient, aided the memory, so he started Rose on PS. Looking for further assistance, Bert brought Rose to the Zucker Hillside Hospital Geriatric Center, but resisted the idea that the available medications may only slow the disease. Not good enough!

When I met Rose and Bert at the Geriatric Center, I immediately saw the emotional pain they were suffering as well as the powerful connection between them. I personally provided support and education, and I encouraged their involvement in groups. In my experience, connecting with others who are dealing with the same disease decreases isolation and enhances coping skills for both the person with the disease and his or her family. Rose, well aware of her memory deficits and saddened by her limitations, joined the early-stage Alzheimer's group. She was amazed by her memory of details of events in her life from long ago. She shared stories from her childhood, her work as a medical secretary, and even recited the preamble to the Constitution.

Despite the frustration of her short-term memory loss, she remains inquisitive about life. Rose is still the Rose she has always been, except that her memory is failing and she must depend more on others. She can no longer drive and, as Bert discovered, can no longer be in a store alone. In 2005, Bert went to the pharmacy to pick up their medicine while Rose looked in another store for a crossword puzzle book. Bert waited outside the store, assuming that Rose was browsing. (Rose certainly looks the same, and it's common for a loved one to forget that the brain is not functioning as it did before.) When Rose did not appear, Bert panicked. She was nowhere to be found. Bert was concerned that even if a kind person found her, Rose would likely give a home address from long ago. Bert called his son, considered calling the police, and circled the area in his car for over an hour. He finally found Rose five blocks away, walking on a major road.

Now she is never out of his sight. Whenever I go to the waiting room to escort Rose and the other members to the group room, Bert asks, "Can I come in?" At first, I explained that the group is only for those with the memory problem. It gives them the freedom to express whatever they need to without concern about their loved one's response. Bert understood. It doesn't stop him, however, from asking every time, "Can I come in?" Now I just say "no" with a smile, and we laugh. He says with a grin, "You can't blame me for trying," and I certainly don't.

Acknowledging his need for support, Bert participates in the caregiver support group. Bert told the group that he stays up at night trying to invent a cure for dementia. He pressures himself and shares this feeling by asking me, "So, have you found a cure yet?" Everyone in the group knows there is none yet, but each one still longs to hear the answer "Yes!" We discuss the research that's currently taking place. But that's not good enough for Bert. He says, "I know there's a cure. I just have to find it."

Bert takes his responsibility to care for Rose seriously. He does admit to being human and sometimes his patience is exhausted by her repetitive questions. For the first several repetitions, Bert answers calmly, but admits to sometimes raising his voice and saying, "You asked me that already." He then experiences feelings of guilt. Rose doesn't remember. It's not her fault. It's the disease. He knows that. The caregiver group members empathize with him. They know what it feels like to love someone and hate the disease that he or she has.

The group members recommend other outlets. These include redirecting her, going into another room, calling a friend, or taking more time alone to recharge. Bert listens, but having more time away from Rose is not his preference. With a great deal of encouragement, Bert allowed Rose to go to an adult day program. At the end of the day, she doesn't remember the activities, but like many with this disease, she remembers the feelings and knows that she had fun. The group members encouraged Bert to increase Rose's attendance at the program, so that he could have more time for himself. Bert, who has spent the past 62 years with Rose, replied, "But what would I do with myself?"

Bert also expresses frustration about Rose moving his papers. He puts something down, and when he looks again, it's not there. He realizes that it's foolish to ask Rose where she put it because she can't remember. He asks her anyway. She says, "I don't remember," and he replies, "It must be the night shift," and begins searching. The important papers are the most upsetting to lose. So I asked Bert if he could put them in a locked drawer or in drawers that Rose does not go through. Bert replied, "She enjoys going through my drawers!" and they both laughed. Rose responded with a sparkle in her eye, "It's true!"

How they love each other. When Bert needed to leave the house for work, he would kiss tissues, and leave each one beautifully folded on the nightstands of his wife and sons' beds so that they would always have his kiss with them. Bert said, "If I could take all of the love songs in the world and condense them into one, that would show the way we feel about one another."

"I love him so much," Rose says.

"You'll get over it!" Bert jokes. They both laugh. A minute later, I start to ask Rose a question. Forgetting that she just told me her feelings, she interrupts and says, "Do you want to know if I love him?"

"Yes," I reply.

"I do...he's my heartbeat."

"Then she'd better take a nitro!" Bert says. A bi m'lacht...they have found a way to laugh again.

Bert is a hero. He has the mind of an engineer and a heart of gold. He would do anything for anyone. But this Mr. Fix-It, with all the love in the world, cannot fix this. What he can do is laugh, and care for his bride. And truly everything he does is for the love of Rose.

Susan Melchione is a licensed clinical social worker and program coordinator of the Neuwirth Memory Disorders Program of the Zucker Hillside Hospital Geriatric Center. She holds a Master of Social Work degree from Adelphi University. For the past 15 years, she has been a direct-care provider to adults and families with neurological disorders, with a specialty in geriatrics.

Part III

Compassion

...brings us to a stop, and for a moment we rise above ourselves.

— *Mason Cooley*

April Showers

Emily Donohue Robbins

We stood together at the edge of the bathtub. My mother had just gotten home from the hospital this April day and her body was too weak to support itself. I lifted her right leg over the tub wall, then her left. She sat down on the folding plastic chair we had wedged into the tub, face lifted up to the water, eyes closed. She told me not to rush her, that she just wanted to sit and feel the water.

My terry-clothed hand rubbed her shoulder blades, around and around, giving birth to soap suds, propelled by the knowledge that it felt good to her. I massaged her scalp with shampoo, not missing one hair on her head. For the 53 years of her life, Patti Robbins loved to shower. She showered through the eight chemo-filled years of her breast cancer: her mastectomy; her multiple rounds of hair loss; her fatigue and vomiting; her radiation and brief remission; the cancer's metastasis to the anus and abdomen; her surgery to implant an external liver drain.

We hesitated when the palliative caregivers suggested that we take her home after several extended hospital stays. Our concerns dissolved when my mother told us that all she wanted to do was to take a shower at home, determined that the cancer would not rob her of her one indulgence. My father rush-ordered three types of shower seats, not knowing which would work best. Anxious to help, I skipped Senior Week celebrations at college, from which I would graduate in three weeks. Watching my mother close her eyes to the shower's tears that April morning, I knew how good it felt for her to rinse everything away.

We hadn't washed her butt; we would wait to do that at the end. When she was ready, I carefully soaped the lump around her anus and even more carefully rinsed the open sores around her vagina. I knew that my mother wanted to preserve her dignity, her privacy; I tried to ease her humiliation. "It's no biggie, Ma," I joked, "I've seen your butt before." When we were done I wrapped her shivering body in dryer-warmed towels.

My mother told me she liked it best when I helped her shower because I didn't rush her as much as everyone else did. I remember feeling then, at 22, like I'd won a prize by being able to give her something no one else could. I told her I had liked it best when she had bathed me as a child, that I'd especially loved it when she splashed in the water from the edge of the bathtub, shaping my soapsuds beard or my brother's mohawk, laughing until we washed away our soapy personas at the showerhead. During this April shower, I wished we were mermaids like we pretended to be when I was young, the bathroom filling with imaginary water, fish swimming gently by us.

After her bath I helped her climb the tub wall and she sat on the toilet to catch her breath. She bound her hair in a towel, twisted like soft serve ice cream. When I handed her the deodorant she lifted her arm, revealing the pea-sized, purple bumps down her side where the cancer had come through her pores. Her dexterity stolen by the neuropathy, she missed her armpit with the stick but I didn't say anything; it didn't matter. She let out an audible "brrrrr" when I unwrapped the towels from around her shoulders. I quickly helped her on with an undershirt—bras didn't matter anymore. I guided her arms into a blue cardigan, the one whose fabric didn't irritate the skin on her arms, and chose socks to match her outfit, just as she always had during the years she had taught kindergarten.

She rested her head on my belly as I stood above her, rubbing her back to make warmth from the friction. I did not rub anywhere near her kidneys, where even the slightest touch hurt her. She exhaled heavily and touched the back of my knee with her right hand. I wished I had warmed more towels for her.

Edema had ballooned her ankles and weighed them down, so after she powdered between her legs, I lifted her left foot into her stretchy cotton pants, and then her right. After a deep breath we got her to her feet, pants up. There was a plastic chair next to the toilet, so she could sit again after dressing. She braced herself on my arms as I took baby steps backward and she followed, like I had followed her when I learned to walk. Careful not to brush the swollen lymph nodes under her arms as I lowered her—"I'm not a baby, you know," she breathed—I stepped away quickly, unsure of how to balance my wanting her to know just how much I had helped and allowing her to think she was still in control. I told her that of course she was not a baby, that I just wanted to help her.

I reached for the dangling bag into which emptied the bile that could no longer drain into her small intestine because a tumor pinched off the connecting duct. The bile stained bright yellow, spotting many of her white cotton nightgowns, so I was careful to hold the bag away from her. The stickiness of it glued the bag stopper shut and I could not twist off the cap. She tried and couldn't open it, either. We had to use pliers to pry open the tube, pointing it downwards into the container where we hoped bile would gush out, because the more bile that drained from her insides, the less leaked into her abdomen. "Two ounces," I told her, as I drained the bag—and we both knew it should have been four. I rinsed the rotten fish smell from the bag, then safety-pinned it to her underwear, a system my mother had invented to keep herself as mobile as possible. I encircled with sterile gauze the base of the tube entering my mother's abdomen. She reminded me to be careful, not to pull or twist, because she was sure her liver could be pulled out. I sealed around the tube with Tegaderm, trimmed neatly so as not to irritate more skin than was already angry with infection.

"Hand me the comb, will you?" she asked, eyes closing, fighting off the pain medication that made her so tired. She brushed her short curls backward, to the left. I asked if she wanted a mirror, she said no. "Do you want to wear earrings?" I asked, as I scanned the framed earring screen we'd painted two summers earlier. The novelty earrings—snowmen, breast cancer ribbons, ladybugs, angels— were surrounded by an array of colorful, stacked-bead earrings, sea glass, and tinted metals. We had made several of the earrings on vacation together. She organized her beads by color and guaranteed we would make a fortune from jewelry making. "How about these?" I asked, taking down her favorite pair, purple and green batik cardboard, and holding them up to her ears. "Only if it's not a hassle," she replied. I had never known her to refuse a pair of earrings; she'd always felt naked without them.

"Let's go sit together, what do you say?" I asked. I ran my fingers through her hair and helped her to her feet, guiding her slowly to the recliner that didn't hurt to sit in. She lowered herself and fell backwards, exhausted. I put her feet up and surrounded her neck with a U-shaped pillow so her head wouldn't loll from side to side. I put the pediatric-sized cannula under her nose so it would breathe oxygen into her tired body. I tucked an unruly curl behind her ear and covered her with two blankets so her cool cleanliness would not chill her.

"You smell so good," I told her after her eyes closed. Something in her throat rose and lowered. She didn't need to say a word to let me to know she was saying thank you.

For months after she died, I thought taking a shower would summon the intimacy of that last vivid memory, but I often felt only sorrow. I would picture her blemished body and wish that I could make more bubbles on her back, soothing her, touching the body in which she was captive, knowing she would have done the same for me.

Sometimes, after I have soaped my body, I sit on the shower floor, curled against the wall, water hot, and cry for my mother. I watch the rivulets of water swirl before they are lost to the darkness of the drain. There is security in the masked sobbing, and the moment is always naked. I have started to use a washcloth, not a loofa, as a small tribute to my mother. I often douse myself in her body spray, reliving her clean smell. These daily ritual changes help me remember how much my mother loved the water, drank the warmth, and how important it is to remember her loving. They help me know that it's okay to have memories so vivid that they hurt, but that I must also remember the memories so vivid that they make me laugh, like the time after a shower she told me to touch her wispy hair because it felt just like "duck fluff."

Now, when I think of the muscles in my mother's neck straining to enjoy her last shower, I think of the peace in her expression: eyes closed, lips drawn, her body capturing the warmth from the water. I think of the time just after her mastectomy that I gave her the black and white poster depicting a young girl who cupped her hands to catch the rain, smiling among her wet curls, captioned "Just as it seems it will never rain again, life comes back."

Emily Donohue Robbins grew up in New Hampshire, where she now works at the Center for Environmental Health Sciences at Dartmouth College. Her mother's eight-year struggle with breast cancer sparked her interest in community health, a subject in which she received a Bachelor of Arts degree from Brown University just four days before her mother died. Emily devotes much of her time to writing about her experiences with her mother's disease and other people's experience with illness; she believes that readers can find courage and inspiration from the stories of others.

Mother-in-Love

Nancy Hoke

"You know about this stuff. I don't." Once again, my husband was struggling to make the best decision he could about his mother's care. Usually, my being a registered nurse was invaluable in making family medical decisions. But now, after many years of helping with both of his parents, it had become more difficult to define my role in all this. Decisions had become more about living and dying than about health.

"Mom, why don't you bring Grandma to your house?" Yet another question from one of our adult daughters, and I began to feel uneasy about an increased pressure my family was trying so hard not to put on me. At one hundred years of age, and widowed for only two years, my mother-in-law still lived in her own home, oblivious to the increasing care she needed. Cancer, surgery, and radiation three years prior had taken their toll on her four-foot-eleven-inch frame, and a gradual progression of dementia was causing frustration. But her will to live independently was as strong as ever.

When I married her only son forty-three years earlier, she had accepted me as a daughter, and my love for her grew as the years passed. For most of her early years, Mother led a life of poverty and frugality. One could not help but love her humble appreciation for living and all she received. Her interest in doing for others came ahead of doing for herself, so it had always been difficult to do things for her, or to give anything to her; sometimes Mother even tried to pay me for her birthday gift. No matter what we said, she always found a way to give some token in return as a thank you.

As she needed more assistance and was less able to do for others, in frustration she expressed anger and resentment toward me. It wasn't her intention, but at times I felt everything I did went either unaccepted or unappreciated. "I'll do it later" was stated in anger, and "I'm not hungry" was her effort to dismiss my plan to fix meals. She saw me as the enemy and often expressed her indignation.

In my head I could understand, but the reality of the struggle eroded the compassion that underlay my giving. At some point, I unconsciously began to measure success in more practical terms: my satisfaction had to come from the act of helping her, not solely from any response Mother gave me. What had been a personal path of care became clinical, and I focused on creating a management plan. One of the wisest decisions in all this came when I told my husband that I would do everything possible for his mother *except* be her primary caregiver. Since I was a nurse, it would have been an easy assumption for both of us to put me in that role, especially because Mother considered me her daughter. However, I was afraid that relationship would be compromised. She would need her son *and* her "daughter," and I wanted to provide comfort more than care.

As Mother became increasingly dependent on our assistance, we made every effort to minimize her losses. She still enjoyed her weekly trips to the grocery store with her son (he joked that she just traded her walker for a grocery cart and could still move fast enough to lose him in the store). While she gradually gave up responsibility for her medication box, she was not about to hand over her washer and dryer to any of us! We tried to help her live independently to the fullest extent of her declining ability, and sometimes she did surprise us with her acceptance of our help.

When we determined Mother would stay in her own home, the challenge we faced centered on her safety. An "alert" necklace was not enough, as she had a fear that if she used it, someone would take her to the hospital and never let her return home. This meant that daily visits were essential. The fifteen-mile round trip became more difficult and longer when the main route underwent major construction for months. I began to wish for a day to myself, some freedom to create my own schedule, some unstructured time to waste and not feel guilty. Then I would wish that I did not *need* to wish for those things. Sometimes none of it made sense, even to me.

Hospice nurses stopped in two or three times each week and aides slowly added days of the week to help her bathe. Mother kept us all entertained with her success in convincing those dedicated individuals that she had bathed herself before they arrived. She maintained her sense of humor only when she felt in charge of her domain, and she remained adamant about who was in charge of her personal care. Our challenge was to provide the care while making it appear to be her idea.

Then one day mother became more confused and took a five-day supply of her medications in one dose. It was clear we could no longer leave her in her home without our providing constant supervision and assistance. At first, Mother was too confused to notice what was being put in place, and I was so busy helping my husband make it happen that it affected my personal feelings very little. Self-examination began to take over, however, and I became more introspective as I lost control over my own life. Before, we had considered her care little more than an inconvenience. Now, we held total responsibility. Our decisions for her care still had everything to do with love, but they were fraught with such necessarily cold practicality that at times the love seemed obscured.

The last nine months of Mother's life became increasingly difficult as we spent long hours at her home. My husband spent nights with her, one of our daughters gave time while her children were in school, and I assumed responsibility to arrange for other help when we were not with her. Soon, our days became all about her calendar. I would be lying to say this came without feelings of despair or resentment, but I knew those feelings were normal and that they would pass. It didn't help to hear her say she was ready to die, that she was not afraid. There were days I wanted the situation to be over, but "over" could only come with her death. I did not want her dead. I just wanted things to be different. Better. She was ready. I wasn't.

Somewhere, somehow, in the middle of these challenges, I changed. I suddenly saw past Mother's physical needs, and was overwhelmed with renewed compassion for her. I had lost life as I knew it, and was already grieving, but I knew I would eventually go on. Mother had lost life as she knew it, and had hope only in death. My overwhelming sadness for her sparked a renewed passion to give meaning to the time that she had left. I felt an intense need to help Mother touch, smell, or hold everything she had loved. It became my mission to bring happiness to her life, and to make her remaining days meaningful. I began to see life through her eyes, and to look for what was truly important.

In the spring, I picked new blossoms for her, realizing this would be the last time she saw the season. She studied the petals, the leaves, and inhaled their fragrance. I put the simplest of bouquets in her favorite containers, and we re-discovered tiny weeds that looked elegant in a dainty porcelain vase. Sometimes my own joy seemed to burst inside me as she smiled. I made sure there was an occasional pie for her to put in the oven, and together we enjoyed the sweet aroma as it baked. My grocery list for her included small potatoes that she could peel, and it helped her to feel that she was still preparing a meal. When she stirred the frying potatoes in butter, the joy I saw and felt was immeasurable. Old photos provided opportunities to revisit friends and family from the past, and laughter was often mixed with tears.

Recent memory loss caused frustration for her, so it became a daily challenge to find items from the past and encourage the telling of a story. I brought her old linens she had made and was humbled as she described the very young woman who had sewn them for her hope chest more than eighty years before. Each day I looked for opportunity to give her as much happiness as possible, and in doing so my own understanding changed. With this growing passion to enrich the end of her life, I found myself becoming a receiver, and a sense of privilege replaced the earlier sense of duty. When she was sad, I felt blessed to sit and hold her as she cried.

One of my most memorable moments came the day she questioned why God let her live.

"Why can't I just die? Why won't He just let me go home?" She sat in her low swivel rocker, and I was on the footstool in front of the chair, holding her hands.

"I don't have an answer, Mother," I said. "But there is one thing I have heard many times and it makes sense to me. They say we are here to learn lessons and to teach lessons to others."

"Well, I don't know why I need to learn any more, and there isn't anything I can teach anyone else."

"Well, Mother, you have taught me so much about how to be a good daughter-in-law, and how to be a good mother-in-law, so maybe that is what you are still doing."

Without a moment's hesitation, she replied, "Well, Nancy, will you please hurry up and learn your lesson so I can go?"

I nearly fell off the stool laughing. However, in that moment I understood how much truth was in that guess about the meaning of life. She *had* been my teacher, and I had modeled much of being an "in-law" after the beautiful example she had set. As I drove home, my eyes still wet from laughter, I cried, thanking God for eyes that saw His lesson in all this.

Three months past her 101st birthday, she finally did make that journey "home." Her final wish had been granted.

It felt strange as I recalled that, months earlier, I had wanted life as it was to end, because the end now proved so painful. I would have missed the opportunity of a lifetime if I had placed my own needs and comfort over hers. Giving all I had for her peace and happiness was not easy; it was not always my first choice. However, it was the right thing to do, and the light it put in her life gave me affirmation of my own purpose. Mother did not know she was the master teacher, but I will forever be grateful for the lessons she taught me by example. Truly, it is in giving that we receive.

Nancy Hoke is the wife of Gene, mother of three daughters, mother-in-law to three "sons," and grandmother of nine. She is a retired registered nurse, former counselor and psychotherapist, and now pursues writing along with volunteer work in her church and community.

(continued from page 78)

More About Hospice

In the United States, hospice is paid through the Medicare Hospice Benefit. Medicare payments account for more than 75% of hospice reimbursements. Medicare requires that recipients spend 80% of hospice care days at home, which means that to qualify for hospice, the patient must have a home and have caregivers (e.g., family members or hired caregivers) capable of providing care. In addition, primarily for financial reasons, Medicare requires that recipients have an estimated survival time of six months or less and that their care be focused on comfort rather than cure. These eligibility rules were created at a time when hospice programs principally served patients with cancer or AIDS, diseases for which the trajectory of dying is relatively predictable. In 1994, for example, 80% of hospice patients had cancer, and the average patient enrolled about one month before death. By 2006, however, only about 40% of hospice patients had cancer. The other leading diagnostic categories include end-stage heart disease, lung disease, kidney or liver failure, neurological illnesses including strokes and dementias, and others. Because hospice increasingly serves patients with such chronic, progressive conditions in which prognostication remains challenging, these eligibility rules now may limit access to care. Asking patients and families to choose between curative care and palliative care is difficult for all concerned and is inconsistent with the current model of care, which views palliative care on a continuum with life-prolonging therapy. Also, this either/or situation may contribute to late referrals and underutilization of hospice services.

Highlights of Hospice

- Embraces all patients coping with advanced illnesses

- Focuses on comfort when cure is not possible

- Emphasizes quality of life

- Promotes personal choice and individual dignity

- Respects the traditions and wishes of the patient and the patient's family

- Most often provides care in the patient's home, but when necessary, can also provide care in the nursing home and inpatient setting

- Uses current treatments and medications appropriate to each individual

- Addresses physical, social, emotional, and spiritual needs

- Provides care and support to the bereaved

(continued on page 127)

Suze Says No

Ned Bastow

"I'm not doing it" were the words that greeted me when I walked into Suze's bedroom to begin her morning routine. I carried a large syringe filled with water to flush my youngest sister's feeding tube, to be followed by anti-nausea medication and ten fluid ounces of a tasteless, high calorie liquid nutrient that had been her only food for the past five months. Afterwards, I would pump in the rest of the morning round of meds meant to stabilize her complicated array of symptoms. We would repeat this process at noon and again at dinner time.

Suze sat on the edge of her bed; she had been waiting for me. "I'm not doing the flush," she declared, "I'm done. I'm not taking the meds, and I'm not taking the food." I stopped dead in my tracks for a moment, then sat beside her on the bed. There was a palpable silence outside the bedroom door, where my wife and my father waited for me to finish the flush before coming in to greet Suze and after which our joint enterprise—caring for Suze— would continue as it had for many days before. I knew they were hanging on every word.

"I've been sitting here for most of the night thinking about this. I don't see any point in it. I just can't do it any longer. Why? What's the point?" This was not the first time Suze had put this question to me, but this time her voice was drained of her characteristic feistiness; what was left sounded of despair mixed with determination.

I had a feeling that Suze had reached this sitting-on-the-side-of-the-bed-all-night decision on my watch, so to speak, because she trusted me to respect her feelings and her decision. She was closer, in age and otherwise, to my brother Bill and my sister Christie, both of whom had been wonderful caregivers for her, but she may have felt that they would pressure her to retreat from her decision.

A lot went through my mind in the few seconds before I answered. I thought about Suze's life—the pain that had occupied much of her 42 years—the crippling, juvenile-onset rheumatoid arthritis; the multiple joint replacements; the plastic knuckles; the rare, chloroquine-induced cardiomyopathy. I thought about her more recent afflictions: three different hospitalizations for pneumonia over the past 18 months; the squamous cell carcinoma at the base of her tongue that left her in too much pain to eat or talk; the radiation and chemotherapy that had pared her down to 70 pounds.

I also thought about how Suze had lived her life: how she never sought or accepted sympathy; how she refused help she didn't absolutely need; how she fought back from every adversity; how she willfully ignored her gnarled hands to become an engineering draftsman, a quilter, and a fine arts photographer.

I also thought about our previous discussions of the "What's the point?" question. I had never presumed to try to answer that question for her. I had told her that these were questions we each had to answer for ourselves. I had always asked her to look back over her life and the people, events, and things that had given her satisfaction and gratification, and which had enriched the lives of others. I told her about my own efforts to answer that question.

All these thoughts swirled about in my head, as well as thoughts about what I felt was my responsibility to the rest of our family and to Suze's many friends. In a way, I felt that I was the representative of the living, that these were defining moments for both of us, and in the face of Suze's determination I knew that I would not be a good representative for the view that life must go on no matter what. At the same time, I couldn't simply say, well, all right, that's the end of that. I turned to face her.

"Suze," I said, "I've learned to be distrustful of decisions made during sleepless nights. Let's think this over. Why don't you start today's meds and food? We can call Michelle (Suze's doctor) and ask her to stop by and visit with us about how things will play out in that scenario, about getting hospice involved, etc. Then, if you still want to go ahead, fine."

She shook her head. I rehashed some of my previous commentary about the "Why?" and "What's the point?" questions, but I knew that those arguments weren't going to carry the day. After about ten minutes of gently pushing back, I accepted what I already knew in my heart: her mind was made up. I told her I would call Michelle and ask her to start the hospice machinery.

I told her I was sure that Dad would support her decision but that she should expect a confrontation with our mother, who I knew would not give in easily. I was half right. Dad told Suze that he would support her decision; he didn't want to see her suffer anymore. But, contrary to my expectation, Mom did not confront Suze and urge (or command) her to choose to live. She told Suze that her decision had her blessing, however reluctantly it was given.

Mom later told us about their conversation. She had tried initially to persuade Suze of the value of life and reminded her about all she had to offer, including this: "Suze, you have excellent taste, and great color sense, and you always give good advice on what people should wear...." Suze wasn't going there. She interrupted quietly, but firmly.

"Wear black."

Mom's first telling of that story, at our late afternoon cocktail hour, brought the house down.

Later that evening, we caregivers had much discussion about Suze's desire to move upstairs and die in her own bedroom, which overlooked Lake Huron's Thunder Bay. Much of our discussion seemed to focus on the convenience of us as caregivers, rather than on Suze. But this was not to be the last word.

The next morning, gathered in the living room, we found we had all, separately, concluded that since this was Suze's dying wish, so to speak, we should honor it. With a "do-it-now" attitude, the whole family walked into the front bedroom and I announced, "Get ready, Suze, we're going to do a Rhett and Scarlett, and I'm going to carry you upstairs." Which I did. She was an unwieldy 70 pounds, and the staircase was very narrow. I was breathing hard when we reached the top, but we made it, and Suze was soon happily ensconced in her own digs.

This turned out to be one of the happiest days in recent memory for Suze. She grooved on virtually everything within her purview: the view of the lake, the smells that wafted through the open window, the feeling of the breeze on her face and arms, all of it. She had a smile on her face for much of the day, the first as it turned out in an 18-day journey to the end of her life with us. But, she was already home.

Ned Bastow grew up in northern Michigan and spent much of his working life in Oklahoma. He retired from the practice of law in 2004 and now lives in Pittsburgh with his wife, Margaret, and an aging Labrador/Beagle mix named Kuma.

The Switch

Sondra Levenson

Margie toddles down the steps toward me, one hand tight on the banister. Under her crooked wig, her eyes peer out from her swollen face. My sister used to be a *fashionista*. A gorgeous woman in her 40s, she ran her errands in Chanel flats and Armani suits. She would paint her eyes with perfect strokes of smoky mascara. But ever since the cancer went to her brain, it's as if a switch has flipped off. She can't judge her own appearance. Today, she's wearing a sweater so tight that her belly pops out beneath its straining fabric. I'm afraid of what will happen once we're on the street. People might stare or whisper about her, or worse, pity her.

"I'm ready," she says.

"Maybe change your sweater?" I suggest, because she shouldn't leave the house with her stomach hanging out, that bare flesh above her slacks.

"No, I look fine," she insists, leaning on the banister. She doesn't want to climb those stairs again, and I can't blame her.

"All right then," I say as we walk out the front door.

In the car, Margie struggles with her seatbelt and I lean over to help her. As I buckle her in, I try to calculate how long it's been since she lost her fashion sense. The last time that Margie really looked like herself—in a cashmere sweater and snug jeans that casually showed off her tush—must have been months ago.

I want her to look good, because the old Margie, the Margie of six months ago, would have been mortified to wear this outfit to a French bistro: a salmon-colored sweater, tight as a sausage casing, matched with green slacks. I'm also worried about Linda, who we're meeting at the restaurant. An old friend of Margie's, she will be shocked and grief-stricken by my sister's sudden decline. More than anything, I want Linda to be cheerful. All week, my sister has been looking forward to this lunch. The last thing she needs is another friend falling apart in front of her.

At the restaurant, the hostess leads us to a table; Margie bobs to her seat; she moves like she's drunk, but no one around us notices, and I think this lunch might go off fine. Then I see Linda at the door, in a tailored business suit, and my heart squeezes. She comes toward us, beaming, and then misses a step. She has noticed Margie's face, the mouth that won't close and the cheeks that seem to be stuffed with marbles. In the last few weeks, Margie has gained twenty pounds from all the steroids.

After a beat, Linda recovers her poise. "Hi ladies," she says. She glides into the booth and sits next to Margie. Linda can't seem to stop clenching and unclenching her hands. But she's smiling at Margie, struggling to make small talk.

"What a cute sweater," she says, her gaze darting away.

Margie orders the Salade nicoise, her favorite. Again I foresee disaster. Margie can't chew anymore.

"The soup is incredible here," I say brightly. "Don't you want that?"

"No, I *like* the salad," she says. Her voice is loud and her inflection makes her sound tipsy. Peeking from behind the menu, Linda looks at me and then at Margie.

I order the soup, sure that I will switch the plates around when they arrive.

"What are the kids doing this summer?" Linda asks. Margie smiles but does not answer. Linda leans forward and repeats the question, louder, realizing that Margie has gone a bit deaf. A woman at the next table studies my sister, as if trying to figure out what's wrong.

Then, thankfully, the waiter arrives with our plates. Margie digs into her salad, puts some lettuce into her mouth, and pockets it in her cheek.

"Good?" I say.

She nods enthusiastically, but then gracefully spits some food into her napkin...and takes another bite. So much for convincing her to eat soup instead—she wants that salad in front of her. She's trying to hang on to what she loves.

When the coffee arrives, Margie and Linda are chatting about their children; it's almost like old times. Margie has become animated. Her blue eyes open wide as she describes her daughter's summer program at UPenn.

Then lunch is over. In the parking lot, Linda gives Margie a kiss on the cheek and walks off. When we drive past her, I notice Linda is shaking her head, her shoulders slumped, and I know she's crying. But my eyes are dry. It's as if a switch has flipped off in my brain too. I don't sob anymore. Instead, I plan a string of pleasures for Margie: a manicurist at her house every Tuesday; a massage therapist on Friday; a bouquet of roses and lilies on Saturday. Margie should enjoy every second she's got left.

We arrive at her house. I unbuckle her seatbelt and we hold hands as we stroll down the path to her front door.

"I'm so tired," she says. When we're in the bedroom, she crawls under one of her favorite blankets.

"It feels so good to be in bed. Do you want to lie down with me?" she asks.

I slip into the other side. We hold hands and watch TV. Above us hangs the crystal chandelier that Margie picked out in better times. The bedside table is crowded with amber pill bottles. I find the sleeping pills and offer her one. I started taking Ambien two years ago, after we learned of the diagnosis. Margie used to rely on sleeping pills too. "Sondra," she would say, "I just need ten more years so I can watch my kids grow up." She was terrified of the final days. Now the final days are here.

She waves away the pills. "I don't need those anymore," she says. And it's true. In the last few weeks, she has become a champion sleeper. She rarely cries or worries about what will happen to her family. She doesn't even ask me if she'll beat the odds. The switch in her brain, the one that turned off her fashion sense, has also shut off her dread. And that has made me feel better too—knowing Margie's emotional suffering has disappeared.

Her breathing falls into a rhythm and I realize she has drifted off. I'm thinking about how the cancer—so cruel in every other away—has been gallant enough to give us these last afternoons, dozing in bed together, talking idly about small things. Margie can't pick out a sweater anymore, and she's lost certain parts of her personality. But she can enjoy lunch and a nap. And right now, I'm grateful for that.

Sondra Levenson lives in Chestnut Hill, Massachusetts, with her husband and two children. She is in the process of writing a memoir, *Half a Life*.

Speaking the Unspoken

Mary Graham

We never talked about why I was there—why I had left training in Europe for a promising career in music and moved back to live with my parents. We never talked about why I had taken only a part-time job, why I sometimes felt compelled to drive home between classes just to chat with Dad for a while. The silence rode through the humdrum days like it always had, as we slept to all the issues that could have been talked about, emotions that could have been felt. The obvious sometimes looms too large to be packed into words.

So I made up unspoken names for myself: names that offered a bit of levity, that defined my role, that told me who I was and gave reason for me being there with Dad in his last months. I was the Breakfast Bringer and the Dinner Dispenser. Dad had aged twenty years since I had last seen him a year before, and he had become absent, wan, and gentle as a grandfather, despite being only fifty-five years old. On occasion, I'd come downstairs to find him trying to cook up an egg on his own, as he had done so capably for decades. Now, egg goo painted the counters, pots decorated the floor and the gas range clicked incessantly, unlit. If I said anything, he'd be insulted, so I'd move around him gently, slipping in some invisible help here and there until he had accomplished a task that made him feel halfway normal again. But most of the time, I'd find him rocking gently in his favorite chair, his glasses cocked at an odd angle on his face, holding a book and staring absently into the distance. Printed sentences had ceased to make sense to him, but he kept trying. He figured that some day the fog in his mind was bound to clear.

My brother had been home to help before I arrived, and it had been a harrowing six months, he reported. Dad was suffering from the emotional stress that came with no longer being able to rely on his own limbs and senses. Along with the physical decline, the chemotherapy had exacerbated Dad's paranoia. Suddenly the door had to be locked against the postman, certain things couldn't be spoken about over the phone because it was tapped, and Dad's valuables had to be hidden, found again, and rehidden in endless cycles. Nonsensical arguments escalated into rash actions. We were convinced Dad would end up dying in an accident rather than from the tumor wreaking havoc in his brain.

I was the Iscador Injector. Iscador is a homeopathic remedy made from mistletoe that is supposed to slow the growth of tumors. From a natural health clinic Dad had attended before my arrival, he had received a large amount of Iscador, and although we weren't certain of its effectiveness at that late stage, we figured it couldn't hurt to keep doing the daily injections. I'd pinch the back of his stiff neck, trying to get a hold of enough to stick the needle into. The illness, together with the medicines, had destroyed his posture. When he paid attention to it, he could straighten up, but the extra attention on the placement of the head, eyebrows raised in a joint effort to keep the heavy globe from sinking, gave the impression of a turtle.

I was the Suspenders Servicer, always ready to put them on or readjust them. While his belly had swelled, his hips had slimmed, and his pants no longer had anything to hang onto. We resorted to suspenders to keep them up. There were several times I had to take on that role, since the suspenders tended to unsnap from his pants when we were out walking on errands. That was dangerous: if even one side came undone, his pants threatened to fall around his ankles.

After breakfast, I became his Personal Singing Coach. Each morning we would do some stretches and movement to keep limber, then sing a set of rounds. Although we each individually loved singing, we had rarely sung together. We both enjoyed singing the simple songs together, although I did feel more like a coach: I pulled and pushed him musically, always attempting to stretch him into places he would not have otherwise gone. But despite my efforts, he gradually ceased being able to hear himself, and would get confused. Knowing it was therapeutic, he stalwartly kept up the daily practice.

My first few weeks back, Dad and I were able to go shopping together; he told the Chaperoning Chauffeur (me) where he wished to go. As time went on, the outings got to be stressful. They entailed finding and putting on the pants with the multiple pockets, filling those pockets with various remedies, a flashlight, emergency items, toiletries, his wallet, glasses and checkbook; fastening the suspenders; finding and putting on shoes that fit his swollen feet; and finding and putting on his favorite soft cap for his balding head. All these items were in perpetual flux–their position in the house shifted constantly, and it was up to the Miracle Memory Machine (me) to keep track of them. This was what made caregiving a full-time job while Dad was still moving through the house on his own. He left a trail of paraphernalia wherever he staggered, and would ask several times an hour where he had left a particular item. The Super Sleuth would remember, find, and deliver it.

I was good at it, but it was not always fun. When the one you are caring for is terminally ill, and his needs spill out around him and crowd into any space you are reserving for yourself, it's difficult to remain constantly obliging. I was not always the Helpful Housekeeper. On one of my whirlwind tours scooping up things that littered the pathways throughout the house, I cleared the space around the chair. I never heard the end of it. "You're just like your mother!" he cried bitterly, complaining about our affliction with the strange disease, Tidyitis. At such times I was the Terrible Tidier, or Papa's Project Preventer.

Even as the decline accelerated and he realized he could no longer get up and down the stairs, we still couldn't talk about the inevitability of the upcoming transition. Sometimes death stands so close, it's too large and too dark for a person to see, and they live in denial of it. While he was in one room searching his file cabinet for everything he needed to apply for jobs the following month when he was certain his mind would clear up and his limbs become more agile, I was in another, leafing through the yellow pages to make necessary arrangements with the local hospice service.

The time came when I named myself Palliative Provider and all other names dropped away. My daily duties were reduced to providing hot packs and morphine for his aches, and glasses of ice cubes to soothe his dry mouth. Stories or prayers often acted as palliatives, too. Or just sitting close by, holding his softened hand. His body had been forced into stillness, but underneath his closed lids, the spirit was restless. I wanted him to stop fighting, stop running. I wanted him to face the shadow, accept its presence. I wanted to become the Surrender Suggester. Someone had to. But sometimes those who are closest are the hardest to speak the truth to–and the hardest to hear it from.

In the end it was the hospice nurse who was allowed to take that title. After a sleepless weekend, I arrived home from work to find the nurse tucking Dad into bed. They both turned to me, and the nurse told me Dad had made the decision. *What decision?*

"You want to tell her?"

"No, you go ahead," Dad sighed wearily, his eyes already closed. The nurse told me he had suggested to Dad that it was time to let go of his body, and asked him if he was ready.

"He said 'yes', so it might be very soon," the nurse said. It was only six hours later that Dad breathed his last.

It's curious, about putting things into words, naming things. Some things can't be spoken, yet some need to be. I could name all the ways I was a caregiver for Dad, in ways he couldn't, just as the hospice nurse had given voice to something I wished I could say, but couldn't. The responsibility for speaking the unspoken is sometimes taken up by another, and we can be grateful for those moments, hoping someday to do the same for others.

Mary Graham was born in Japan and has traveled extensively throughout her life. She graduated from Middlebury College and is now a freelance writer living in Vermont.

Taking Care of Ellie
Maria V. Ciletti

The waiting room of St. Joseph's oncology department was packed almost to standing room only. This was our third visit to the oncologist this week. What had started out as a routine visit, six weeks ago, had become a full-out effort to battle a firestorm of metastasizing cancer cells.

A woman wearing a pink and white polyester track suit and a pink turban sat down next to me and my aunt, Ellie. The woman was thin and jaundiced; an obvious sign that her cancer had already reached her liver. Oxygen hissed through the plastic cannula in her nose from a portable unit, a small silver torpedo she carried like a shoulder purse. Aunt Ellie looked up from her *Woman's Day* magazine, smiled at the woman, and said hello.

Ellie, like most of the ladies in the waiting room, also wore a turban to hide her patchy hair, one of the lovely side effects that the cancer treatments had bestowed on them. As Ellie and the woman waited to be seen by the doctor, they exchanged war stories of their illnesses. The two women talked like they were schoolkids meeting up for the first day of class. The woman in the pink turban had lung cancer. "Worked forty years as a waitress at Mickey's Diner and never smoked a cigarette in my life," she said, her voice raspy as if she had smoked three packs of unfiltered Pall Malls a day.

Aunt Ellie had breast cancer. She went on to tell the woman that the original tumor was discovered during her yearly mammogram and that she had been in remission for seven years. But her last bone scan had turned up several "hot spots." After exchanging their health information, the two women went on to discuss a peach cobbler recipe Ellie had found in the *Woman's Day* magazine like it was a normal thing to be exchanging recipes while chemotherapy drugs flowed through their veins.

This visit turned out to be an especially hard one for us. Ellie's doctor told us that all the aggressive chemotherapy she had been receiving for the past six weeks had done nothing to stop her tumor from spreading. He said that her CAT scan from yesterday showed that cancer had not only spread to her liver and lung, but to her pancreas as well. He also told her there was nothing more that could be done and to go home and put her affairs in order and make the best of the time she had left.

After the doctor left, Ellie sat on the exam table with her hands folded in her lap, quiet. I am sure she was unable to believe that there really was no hope. She had done all the things they told her to do. She had endured hours of chemotherapy and day after day of nausea and vomiting and bone pain. She had intravenous ports inserted under her skin because all the veins in her hands and arms were shot. She took her medication meticulously and now they were telling her there was nothing more they could do. That seemed so unfair.

The next step was to take Ellie home and prepare her for what remained. In spite of our offers to have her stay with us, she insisted on staying in her own home. We invested in a Life Call system for Ellie to use when we weren't there. Under much protest from Ellie, hospice was called in. Within a few hours a hospital bed and oxygen were delivered and a hospice nurse was at the house filling out intake forms and asking a lot of questions no one wanted to answer.

"Miss Ciletti, if your heart should stop or if you stop breathing, do you want us to do CPR?"

"My niece will do it," Aunt Ellie answered. "She's a nurse. If I need anything she will do it."

Her comment made me laugh. Thinking she may not have understood the nurse's question, I said, "Ellie, she means if I'm not here...do you want them to do CPR?"

"I don't need them here. What do I need them for if I have you?" she said.

The hospice nurse looked up at me partly with frustration and partly with understanding. She went on to the next question.

"Miss Ciletti, do you live alone here?"

Ellie nodded.

"You do realize that at some point you won't be able to stay here by yourself. We have an inpatient facility you are welcome to stay at when that time comes."

Ellie shifted in her chair. "Look," she said. "I was born in this house and I'll die here too. I appreciate what you are trying to do, but I'm okay. Thank you anyway."

The hospice nurse looked up at me again. I shrugged my shoulders knowing all too well she wasn't going to get anywhere with Ellie. After all, Ellie was the most independent among her five sisters and I am sure she would carry that distinction to the very end.

Ellie fought for several weeks, still unwilling to admit that hope was lost. But as time went on, she got weaker and weaker to the point where even she couldn't ignore the inevitable. Eventually, we took shifts staying with Ellie. Aunt Lou, Ellie's oldest sister, stayed with Ellie during the day and my partner, Rose, and I would stay in the evening and during the night, when Ellie would let us. "What are you gonna do," Ellie would ask, "sit up all night and watch me sleep?" She'd insist we go home and get some rest, adding, "You look like crap." I took her insults as backdoor thank yous.

After work each evening Rose and I would go to Ellie's house and sit with her and watch Cleveland Indians baseball games and DVD's of *Mr. Ed*, her favorite TV show. I'd make her tea and toast and she'd pretend to eat it more for my benefit than hers. When she got tired, she'd ask me to take her to bed. I'd shuffle behind her, this woman who at one time could really cut a rug, as she struggled to walk to her tiny bedroom, the same room in which she was born.

Bedtime got earlier and earlier and soon she was asking to go to bed at six in the evening. She had lost interest in the baseball games. Even Mr. Ed couldn't make her laugh anymore.

One evening as I was putting her to bed she started to cry. I sat down next to her on the bed.

"Rough day, huh?" I asked.

She nodded, tears brimming in her eyes.

"You want to talk about it?"

She lowered her head and gave no response. I took her boney hands into mine and tried to rub some warmth into them—these were the same hands that held cards while playing Crazy Eights with my brother and me (she let us win every time), and the same hands that made light bulbs at the General Electric plant for over thirty years.

"You know Ellie, there is nothing you can't tell me," I said. "I've seen it all and heard it all. Nothing you say will hurt me or scare me."

Ellie looked up. Her eyes locked on mine and her lips quivered. "I'm ready to go, Ree," she said, barely getting the words out.

They hit me like a ton of bricks. But I knew I had to be strong for her. "It's okay to let go," I said. Now I was having trouble getting the words out. "I'm gonna miss you, Ellie," I said. "You have been such a big part of my life. But I understand it's time."

I hugged her tight and we both started to cry. I wiped her tears away with my hand. We talked for a while, Ellie stoically giving me the necessary information regarding her legal matters, burial preference, and how she wanted things done. I promised her I would make sure her wishes were carried out. She asked me to tell my brother and sister and Rose her wishes. I told her I would.

Ellie hung on for two weeks after that conversation. Rose and I slept on the living room floor each night and day by day Ellie got weaker and more disoriented. She stopped eating altogether and slept most of the time.

In those final days, Ellie didn't want much company. She was very particular about whom she wanted around her and whom she didn't. She loved having my sister's kids at the house. I would watch her as she looked at them intensely, trying to memorize their beautiful young faces.

With me, my brother, and my partner Rose at her bedside on a rainy Sunday evening, Elvira Delores Ciletti left this world. Ellie was a champion in the way she fought her disease. She handled things her way and with dignity. She will always be my hero.

This journey with Ellie was one of the most difficult I have ever made, but I am thankful for the opportunity to have taken it with her. I don't think you can get any closer to someone than when you share this kind of experience with them. And in doing so, you are giving your loved one the greatest gift ever: unconditional love. And we all can use a little more of that.

Maria V. Ciletti is a registered nurse working as a medical administrator for a family practice in Niles, Ohio. She graduated from Choffin School of Practical Nursing in 1982 and Sharon General Hospital School of Nursing in 1987. She did her undergraduate studies at Youngstown State University. She currently lives in Niles, Ohio, with her partner, Rose.

(continued from page 106)

How and When Does Hospice Start?

Anyone can inquire about hospice services. A patient or a loved one may call a local hospice and request services. The hospice staff will then contact the patient's physician to determine if a referral to hospice is appropriate. Another way to inquire about hospice is for the patient to talk with his or her physician, and the physician can make a referral to hospice.

Hospice can begin as soon as a referral is made by the person's doctor. The hospice staff will then contact the person referred to set up an initial meeting to review the services the hospice will offer and sign the necessary consent forms for care to begin. Usually, care is ready to begin within a day or two of a referral. However, in urgent situations, service may begin sooner.

When Is the Right Time to Ask About Hospice?

Now is the best time to learn more about hospice care and ask questions about what to expect. Although end-of-life care may be difficult to discuss, it is best for loved ones and family members to share their wishes long before it becomes a concern. This can greatly reduce stress when the time for hospice becomes apparent. By having these discussions in advance, uncomfortable situations can be avoided. Instead, educated decisions can be made that include the advice and input of loved ones. As the adage goes, "knowledge is power." The comment of one of my most memorable hospice patients, a 67-year-old lobbyist with ovarian cancer, emphasizes advance planning and achieving closure. She said humorously, "I'd rather sit shiva while I am still alive."

Choosing a Hospice

There may be one hospice organization or several that serve a person's community. It is important to find out about the services that each hospice offers. If there are several hospices that serve your area, you may want to request services from a particular hospice and can communicate that wish to your physician. Some common questions from individuals and loved ones facing life-limiting illnesses include:

- Are all hospices the same?

- How do I decide if hospice is the appropriate care choice for me?

- How do I choose among different hospice programs?

- If there is only one hospice program in my community, how do I determine if it is a good one?

Not all hospices are the same. Not-for-profit hospice programs may differ from for-profit programs in their ultimate priorities. Hospices with full-time, multiple, or dedicated medical directors likely provide stronger medical support and medical home visits. Hospices with larger patient populations (with an average census of greater than 200 per day) are more likely to provide "open access"— accepting patients with more expensive medications or providing palliative radiation therapy, for example.

Determining if a hospice is right for you may best be learned by calling different hospices and asking them about their services. It is a good idea to talk to people you trust who work in healthcare or aging services or who have received support from a hospice, such as physicians, nurses, or other healthcare professionals, social workers, your clergyman, or friends or neighbors who have direct experience with hospice care.

(continued on page 137)

Assessment Number Two

Maryann Lesert

Gina, Lou and I are sitting at the kitchen table, having coffee. Dad is outside, puttering around the shed. It's a very windy spring day. Lou and I had arrived to tell Dad that someone named Fran was coming over to do a "senior health assessment"; Gina, sounding winded, greeted us in the driveway. "Your Dad's out back trying to get himself blown away along with the shed."

We walked to the cleared-out garage. Dad walked in, pointing at us with his middle finger, as he's always done. "Good, good. You're here to help. That door," he said, "the wind just took it and wham!"

He went to his workbench, fumbling with a spread of tools: a wrench, some washers, an assortment of screwdrivers and nails. But he couldn't find the hammer—I figured Gina had hidden it from him. I watched Dad pick up and set down tool after tool, as if wanting his hands to tell him which one was right. "He didn't set the hook on the door, and it got blown open too hard," Gina told us.

The last time I visited, Dad was trying to fix the sprinklers, which, for some reason, meant he had to cut the hose to the water heater. Now Dad found a handsaw. "Oh no-ho-ho, don't you take that out there," Gina scolded. "Come on. Come and have coffee. The girls are here."

In the kitchen, as Gina warmed the morning coffee in the microwave, Dad stood, glancing out the window, shifting his weight from foot to foot as he often did when fixated on something and wanting to get to it. I put my hands on his shoulders and told him the wind was too strong to work outside. But as soon as the coffee was poured and he couldn't figure out where to sit, he was out the back door. Gina hollered after him, too tired to chase him, "Lee, don't you dare nail anything on that shed!"

The three of us talk now, preparing for questions Dad will be asked about eating, dressing, and showering. He's been struggling with shirts, doing odd things with the sleeves as he tries to put them on. Sweatshirts, Gina says, work best.

Curious to see what Dad is doing, I get up from the table and go to the window. I should be helping, as Lou tries to elicit the response we need from Gina about when she wants us to move him, but I stand, fascinated, watching Dad try to "fix" the shed. He's holding a piece of molding in his hands, trying to make it fit in some magic, matching place. It's not the complete lack of his spatial awareness that fascinates me, but rather the mystery of what must be going on in his mind as he stands before the open doorway of the shed, unable to decipher the spaces and shapes before him. First he places the thin strip of wood across the opening on a diagonal. The molding doesn't reach to the other side. He toddles to one corner of the shed and holds the strip of wood flush to its edge. When that doesn't work, he moves to the other side of the shed and puts the board flush with that corner. I watch as he repeatedly slides it up and down. But the board is too short, so he reaches overhead and places the board under the roof line, extending it downward towards the open doorway. What is happening in his mind when he does these things?

"You guys ought to come and see this, how he's trying to make the molding fit," I say. Lou and Gina stare back at me, blankly, wondering how I can find this interesting. "I know," I say, "but it's fascinating, in a way, watching as he tries to fit the shape." Gina looks tired. Lou looks at me with one eyebrow raised, beaming "Shut up" into my eyes.

Dad is trying to place the molding parallel to the angle of the roof now. Only instead of tucking the board up under the roof slant, he positions the board diagonally across the opening. But the double-door opening is too wide.

I want Gina and Lou to see what I see. Gina just smiles tiredly at Dad's antics and my sense of wonder. Lou's eyes are telling me to be more sensitive to how exasperating it is for Gina to live with a man with whom she once traveled the world, but who is now in her backyard trying to fit a piece of molding in all sorts of wildly impossible positions on the shed. But I can't attend to their need for camaraderie. I can only watch. So I apologize. "I know it's sad. I do. But I can't help it. It's so interesting to watch the process."

"I'm sure it is," Lou says, eyeing me hard, "when you don't spend every waking minute with the person."

I try to narrate what Dad is doing, but Lou and Gina ignore me, talking to each other about the upcoming health assessment. Gina isn't ready to talk "assisted living" with Dad. "Not quite yet," she says, so for now we're telling him that these in-home visits which Lou and I have arranged are standard for seniors like Dad, to see if he might benefit from services such as an emergency call box or meals on wheels.

Last week's assessment with Shelley, the Director of Care of our second-choice assisted living facility, did not go well. With French-manicured nails and a frilly V-neck dress, she didn't look like any nurses I know. Shelley asked Dad direct questions: "How do you do with dressing yourself? Any problems with buttons or shoes?" Dad grew quiet, sitting with his hands clasped in his lap, nodding and smiling uncomfortably. Shelley wrote in codes, "AE30" and

"I-15" in boxes on a preprinted form. Later, when Lou made me call and ask Shelley what assessment form she was using, Shelley said it came from "property management."

Lou is pressing Gina for answers now. "Gina," Lou says, in her objective voice, the one that means she's organizing, "I'm going to ask you something directly and I want you to answer honestly, whatever you feel." Lou is younger than I am, but this look— along with hands out before her, directing, mouth set—says to me, Back off, I'm handling it. She was Daddy's girl. "If we find a place for him, we're assuming you want us to do this soon. Is that what you want?" I keep my eyes on Dad. He's returned to the corners of the shed, shifting left then right, placing the molding flush with one corner, then the other. But he keeps coming back to a faded shape along the right edge of the doorway.

"If he wants it," Gina answers.

Lou sighs. "Let me rephrase that. That wasn't fair." Lou sounds legal. That's what bugs me. But these are difficult words, and she hates confrontation. "Okay, how soon do you want us to do this?"

Gina hesitates, her "ho-ho-ho" barely audible as a break in her breath. "I don't know (ho-ho)...I don't want to hurt him."

Dad is back to that shadow of faded paint along the edge of the doorway, which represents where the piece of wood in Dad's hand had fitted to the shed. Dad is sliding the molding up and down, parallel to the ground, when it needs to be perpendicular.

A year ago, we were disturbed by his "visions." I borrowed his car to drive to a workshop in Louisville last spring, and he called me several times to warn me about a leak in one of the hoses. By the time he'd called a fourth and fifth time, I envisioned a Medusa of hoses being unleashed from under the hood. "They'll come right out and pop your hood," he told me. "And the oil. You just can't believe the oil. They'll get to spraying it so thick, hoses everywhere, just a-thrashing, and you can't see a thing." Then there was the respiratory virus he caught over the winter. He'd tell us how his lungs were just "slap, slap, slapping" against his chest when he coughed, and sometimes, one of his lungs would "slap right out his back with the waterfall." Gina decided, finally, that she could not care for him any longer when he woke her up in the middle of the night and said, "Gina...I forgot how to go to the bathroom."

Lou is telling Gina about Fran, the director of our first-choice assisted living facility, who is due any minute. Fran's nails, she said, are short and she has the hands of a nurse: well-used, often-washed, and slightly red. When we visited Fran's facility and asked questions about licensing and staff ratios and training, she smiled and understood. "It's like trying to find good childcare, isn't it," she said. Fran is a degreed registered nurse. Shelley, with her polished nails (forgive me), is a licensed practical nurse. An LPN directing care?

I'm trying to leave Gina and Lou to their more serious talk. I think Dad is about to get it. He's back to that strip of faded paint along the edge of the doorway, and he's placed the molding upright, nearby. A few slides and he'll have it.

"Hah! I think he's got it."

Gina must have already seen this played out a hundred times, because she stands up, moves to the window, slides it open, and hollers. "Lee! It doesn't belong there! It belongs on the door!"

She grumbles as she sits. "It's got to go on the door, it's the inside piece that fits on the door."

Thankfully, Dad doesn't have the door. I stand and watch as Dad, distracted, holds the molding on an angle again, and moves toward open space.

I want to "shush" Gina. Redirect, never correct, as Fran would say. He almost had it. But my eyes fill with tears, and I decide to be thankful. Gina is exhausted, and I should be happy to have these moments to watch, so I apologize. "I'm sorry."

"I know," she smiles, "I know, Hon." And with that Gina is up again, rising from the chair and reaching out to widen the open casement window in one motion, as if she's done this so many times that it is an automatic, physical reaction to her sense of frustration. "Lee! Get in here and have coffee with your daughters!"

Gina is living minute by minute with the mechanics of Dad's memory loss. A year ago, we sat in a specialist's office, amazed that Dad could no longer tell time or draw a box or sign his name. Now she's living with a man she accompanies more as a "sitter" than a girlfriend. Dad has lived with Gina for ten years, here in this house where Gina had already taken care of one dying man, her husband of four decades, before she and Dad gave each other rings but decided not to go through a marriage ceremony and all the legalities. Gina can't do it all again. Dad's doctor, in our most recent consultation, called Gina Dad's "umbilical cord." But he warned us that Gina's blood pressure, with her lack of sleep and all the anxiety, was reaching dangerously high levels. It was time for Gina to care for herself.

Back inside, Dad stands away from the table with his coffee cup. He looks young still, even at seventy-six. His dark hair is graying, and he's bald on top, but he has been for years. Up until this year, he was still playing "old-guy" softball. Sure, his teammates had to correct his stance at the plate and remind him which base to run to and when to put his glove on, but he was out there, enjoying the game. This year, the coach asked Gina not to sign him up. Now he cannot be left alone, not for a minute, it seems. He is waking up in the middle of the night, telling Gina he wants to go home.

Dad turns to go outside, but something about the dining room window catches his eye, and he moves toward it. The casing is open farther than the sliding storm window, which, just moments ago, Gina pulled back so she could lean out and wave him in; I can tell he doesn't like the relationship between these shapes. Can't something fit? He tinkers with the heavy wooden casing and the inner storm window, sliding them back and forth. It's just like one of the social workers said, "There's no sense in correcting them when they get fixated on something, they're trying to find closure."

As I watch Dad strive for some success with shapes, I can't stop feeling there's a map to it, a particular puzzle or pathway for each person; I can see Dad's. He's always been a fix-it person. Always. And when there were no standards or models to follow, he made up his own—like the homemade sheet metal monster of a snow sled he made that we called the Blue Whale, the one that trapped us under its weight when it capsized on the edge of a snow bank and our legs flailed for the new home movie camera as Mom, behind the lens, laughed until she cried. Or the new floorboards Dad soldered and bolted under the driver's seat of Lou's rusting old Nova. I get goose bumps watching him, thinking that for everyone, and for Dad, too, there must be some neural pathway that misfires and reroutes in ways that correlate to how that person used their brain all along. And I wish, so fiercely sometimes, that we had more time to slow down and watch and listen. To take note. In so many ways, I wish we simply had more time.

But Fran is coming; Fran with the hands of a nurse. Fran and her facility, with four wide-open wings and wardrobe closets with white linings—no hallways or dark closets. But Fran's facility doesn't have showers in the rooms. Dad would have to make his way to the end of his wing, carrying a drawstring clothing bag. And soon, they may not let him shower on his own. But this is a silly detail to get hung up on, isn't it?

Dad has been waiting; I can feel it, for me to look at him, that same gradual awareness I used to feel when the kids were small and they'd shuffle and stare and wait for me to notice them. He catches my eye and he points, with his middle finger, toward the window. There, he communicates with a huge, triangular smile. Hah-hah! There. I got it. After much tinkering, he has positioned the window casing and the inner screen so that they line up exactly. Exactly.

There. I say to myself, nodding in his direction. There. For now, one piece fits.

Maryann Lesert's award-winning plays include *The Music in the Mess*, *Samhain* and *Natural Causes*, a finalist for the Princess Grace Foundation's National Playwright fellowship. Her first novel, *Base Ten*, was written while she earned a master's degree in fine arts in fiction from Spalding University. This story is an excerpt from her current novel-in-progress, a work that draws upon her real-life experiences with her father's Alzheimer's disease. She lives in Michigan.

(continued from page 128)

Questions to Ask When Choosing a Hospice Program

- How long does it typically take the hospice to enroll someone once the request for services is made?

- What services are provided?

- What kind of support is available to the family/caregiver?

- What roles do the attending physician and hospice play?

- What does the hospice volunteer do?

- How does hospice work to keep the patient comfortable?

- How are services provided after hours?

- How and where does hospice provide short-term inpatient care?

- With which nursing homes or long-term care facilities does the hospice work?

- How are hospices services paid for?

- Can I still see my own doctor? How would that work?

(continued on page 158)

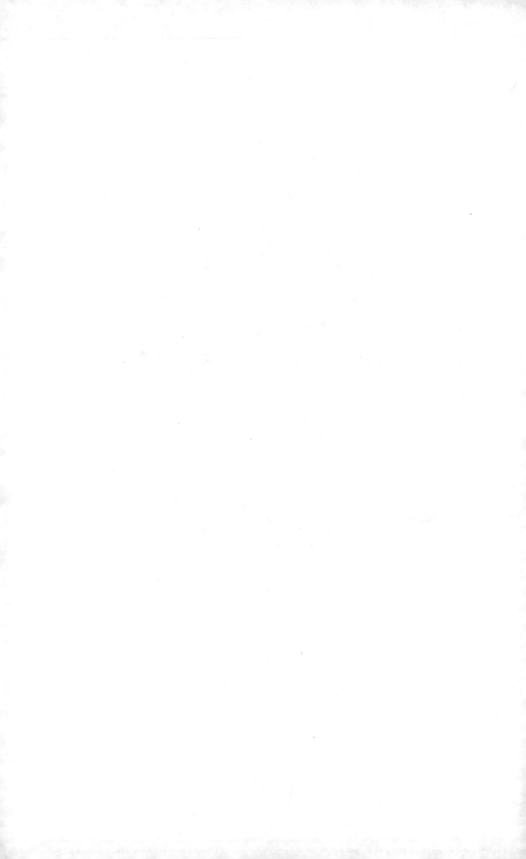

Part IV
Patience

...is one of the most-used tools in the caregiver's toolkit.

Give Caring

Joanne Hirase-Stacey

I am slowly learning to have patience with my patients. I've been thrust into a role I wasn't prepared to play, or even contemplated having to play. After all, Mom and Dad had always been healthy, save for the stroke Dad had in 1993. But at ages 76 and 80 respectively, they've turned that corner from nurturing to needing, and as an only child, the responsibility has fallen on my shoulders. This isn't to say I'm not up for the task, or am refusing to care for them. Not at all. I just didn't think it would be so hard, especially with people I love.

It started off easily enough, when Mom was admitted into the hospital with pneumonia. I live a couple of hours away from them, so I took up residence on the couch since my old bedroom is now the TV room. Dad said he was going to be a new man and be more helpful around the house. I soon discovered that what he said and what he does are not the same.

"Dad, it's Monday, vacuuming day."

"Why don't you do it?"

"It's your job now."

"I don't want it."

Then:

"Dad, don't forget to water the plants."

"You do it."

"It's your job."

"I don't want it."

And so on.

When we finally got Mom home, she was incapable of doing much besides sitting, so she was very appreciative of the help. But little by little, as her health started improving, she became resentful. When Dad fell down the stairs, we found out he'd had a mini-stroke.

"He's just mad because I'm getting all the attention."

"No, he really had a minor stroke."

"He's just saying that so I have to take care of him when he should take care of me."

And it didn't stop there:

"Dad doesn't feed me."

"That's because I told him not to. You have to start doing some things for yourself."

"He doesn't do anything but sit in front of the television."

"Neither do you."

Thus, the daily battles began with her as well.

Even though it was the dead of winter and the temperatures were unusually low, I ran almost every day. It was my respite, my time to myself where everything was fine and life was back to whatever normalcy I had before. The neighbors and the home health-care aides and nurses thought I was crazy. That is definitely the road I was headed for, so I kept running—in a different direction.

Every day, in the bone-chilling cold, I pondered the same thing: *What happened to the robust, lively, rational folks I knew? Now they're temperamental, stubborn, tantrum throwing people.* I realized it's the dreaded role reversal, so clichéd but true. Then I came down hard on myself: *How can I begrudge the past few months of care when they've had to put up with me and my wild antics for years?*

"I'm a terrible person, not a good caregiver," I lamented to my husband. "I feel guilty about being so hard on them."

"You're fine. You're just being you."

That didn't make me feel any better.

One particularly brisk morning, I finally had the epiphany I'd been waiting for. I ran around a corner, and there was a man on his porch smoking a cigarette, jumping up and down to keep warm. He looked at me like I was nuts for purposely being out in the cold to run. I looked at him like he was nuts for needing a cigarette so badly he'd risk frostbite on his lips. But at that moment, I knew. I knew my frustration and annoyance were my problem and caused by my attitude, not by anyone else. It was my choice. I choose to run and not to smoke, he chooses to smoke and not to run. I choose to be frustrated and annoyed, but no one is choosing to frustrate and annoy me.

After this clarity of reason, I also realized "caregiving" is easy, but what I call "give caring" is not. There is a difference: caregiving involves the day-to-day monotonous activities that are necessary, such as making sure medications are taken, that they eat and bathe. Give caring happens every time I am caring but choose not to be aggravated.

The evolution to better give caring is painful, but I'm getting to the point where I don't verbalize how much dog hair is missed when Dad finally gets around to vacuuming. It annoys me, but only when I choose to let it. I try not to get frustrated at how slow they walk, or how long it takes them to eat, or how set they are in their ways. I am constantly adjusting my attitude to give caring so I can have a happier balance. There are still many moments when I have to rewind and think of a more appropriate thing I should have said than whatever impatient words flew out of my mouth. But my new mantra, "think then talk" or "TTT", is starting to take over.

My new role took on an interesting twist when I noticed Mom's memory going haywire. Unfortunately for her, but fortunately for me, it's provided some comic relief. I got out a puzzle, hoping it would help with brain function. She happily looked for the edge pieces and when she found one, put it into the puzzle box lid. After about an hour of searching, she went to the bathroom. When she came out minutes later, she saw the pieces on the table and said, "Oh look, a puzzle. I love puzzles!" I do my best not to laugh at these episodes, and I try to wait until I'm pretty sure she can't hear me. Dad just stares at her, shakes his head, and walks away.

Since my epiphany, I've spoken to many caregivers and explained my theory on give caring. I'm amazed how many people tell me they have the same struggles and are glad they're not the only ones feeling the same way, even those who I think are remarkable at give caring. I still have a long way to go in my battle to be good at give caring, but I think I'm on the right path. I rejoice in knowing I'm not alone, but can always find others who empathize with me.

Joanne Hirase-Stacey is a corporate attorney in the semiconductor business who lives with her husband and dogs in southeastern Idaho. She has had short stories published in *The Storyteller* and *Thema* and will be published in *The Upper Room* and *Dog Blessings* in 2008. Joanne is working on her first novel.

Postpartum Blues Plus Twenty
Claire Luna-Pinsker

Is it possible to have postpartum depression for over twenty years? I consider myself the first diagnosed case.

I adore my youngest son, my Christmas gift, a baby I begged my ex-husband for. Mothering him is draining me now that I'm older. For how much longer will I need to remind him (he's 20 now) to jump in the shower? It's a standard message I repeat over and over, otherwise he'll remain in pajamas. I long to do the same, which is why I realize I'm suffering an extended period of postpartum depression. My son has Asperger's syndrome. Thankfully, he doesn't have a total noncommunicative form of autism, but his disorder places a real strain on me as his main caregiver. My children are my heart and I'd gladly surrender my life for them, but there are times when I feel like I will be sucked dry by the relentless demands of an autistic child.

During my pregnancy, I realized he was going to be different. In utero he never rested, always twisting and turning, karate chopping painfully against my stomach. My abdomen stretched to an enormous size until, on Christmas Eve, he entered the world weighing in at ten pounds and six ounces. He nursed in a matter of seconds, constantly squirming, his roaming eyes taking in the entire world. My nickname for him was Panoramic Baby.

My Panoramic Baby wouldn't cuddle and complained if swaddled, preferring to lie alone on a blanket or catnap in a baby swing. In his toddler years, when disturbing symptoms intensified, I couldn't turn my back on him. Child-protective devices were useless; he managed to maneuver his way around them like an escape artist.

Once I took him shopping with me, a harness zipped up his back because he wouldn't stay in a stroller. People gawked, but I felt he was safe, connected to me. While I looked through clothing, his strap safely secured around my wrist, he scurried underneath the rack. As I stepped after him, the leash went taut and almost broke my wrist. Following the leash, I found an empty harness zipped securely around a pole, and my son nowhere to be seen. He had escaped in a matter of seconds.

Panic-stricken, I screamed his name, rushing around, peering underneath other racks. *What kind of irresponsible mother am I*, I thought. Luckily, another mother found him (as he was about to get on the escalator), and took him to security. And there he sat, talking a mile a minute to a guard. His calm greeting was, "Hi Mommy." A con artist could learn something by observing my son's amazing capacity to outwit you.

When he was five I decided, after experiencing two frantic years of nursery school, that kindergarten was the answer to stimulate his mind and to harness his overactive brain energy. On the first day of school I wrote his teacher a note:

Dear Teacher,

Here's my heaven-sent child. He's now in your expert hands. Please don't take your eyes off him for a second. He requires strict supervision and I do pay my school taxes! Please send my son home exhausted!

As he grew older, new problems emerged. A big one was autistic rage. No one has figured out how to switch off autistic rage before it inevitably escalates. Once, I was rudely awakened at two in the morning by repetitive popping sounds, as if firecrackers were exploding in my house. The sound emanated from a broken speaker in his stereo system. I decided to calmly discuss the situation with him over lunch the next day, and requested that he disconnect the broken speaker because it was disturbing my sleep. Continuing to eat, he replied with a few grunts, his usual pattern of speech. When I asked for eye contact, an open bottle of ketchup whizzed past my ear, landing on the living room carpet, spraying the entire area. Then a container of fruit punch slammed against my kitchen wall. Before I could respond, kitchen chairs were knocked over as he stomped upstairs, kicking open his bedroom door, his foot splintering the wood panel. This was followed by a stream of cursing before his door slammed shut.

I was momentarily stunned by this outburst. I might have reacted by flying upstairs, kicking open his door and grabbing him by the neck and saying, "I brought you into this world and I'll take you out. Who do you think you are, destroying my home?" But this, of course, was an imagined reaction because I'm the mature individual who has to maintain complete control. Instead, hot flashes consumed me and, perspiring, I grabbed a bottle of carpet cleaner from a well-stocked cabinet. Struggling to the floor on arthritic knees, I scrubbed frantically at ketchup streaks. He sat in his room cooling down, with his popping surround sound system on full blast while I mentally planned placement in a group home, venting, unable to initiate this final step because I'm "Super Mom."

Later on, calmly apologizing for the millionth time, he robotically recited the correct way to manage rage, learned from attending a six-week anger management class. With a photographic memory he recalled exactly the appropriate words. As we scrubbed the walls together, he broke the tension by remarking dryly, "You can't even see where the ketchup landed."

People on the outside looking in might not be able to see humor in some of the dire situations my son's autism has caused; my sometimes warped sense of humor keeps me going. I once envisioned that my life would, eventually, be a total breeze and looked forward to being an empty nester, never imagining that I'd still be frantically trying to secure a babysitter for a two hundred pound twenty-year-old just to escape for a weekend. Over the years, my life has evolved to where I plan nothing without considering him first. I spend endless hours researching autism, reading everything I can get my hands on, continuing education on the latest developments. I speak to doctors, psychologists, psychiatrists, attend group therapies, and maintain direct contact with schools. Fortunately, his schools have been fantastic, willing to attempt anything to assist my challenged son. And he challenges them with his amazing wit, eagerness to learn and remarkable gift for soaking up knowledge.

During the past four years he's developed physically into a man, maturing to function in most classroom situations without supervision, using his own methods to overcome problems hindering him. If you notice him you'll see an adolescent suffering from acne, with a slightly awkward gait, kinetic eye movements and hand tremors. You probably wouldn't give him a second glance, but for him every day is a struggle to control the impulses his brain puts out. Literal in thought, with a wry sense of humor, his greatest personality trait is a strong sense of self-esteem. And no matter what happens, he's never depressed. In some ways it's a marvelous way to live, waking up and going to bed happy.

He's a young man attending community college for a degree in electronics, afterwards returning home and retreating into his bedroom. With no friends and no interest in making any, he's content to watch hours of television and be on his computer. His favorite phrase is, "I'm busy." He manages to write college-level essays, create elaborate websites and converse with friends in cyberspace. To explain in detail, face to face, what he's doing is an impossible task for him. Emotionally and socially he's way behind his peers, still reacting childishly and impulsively, taking enough medication to sedate a horse. Thankfully, they ease some of his symptoms and they are taken willingly. Only once did I discover a collection of his medications, hidden underneath his pillow. An increase in his symptoms clued me in within a few days. His reasoning: "I think I'm better now. I don't need them." Self-medication permission was abruptly taken away.

There apparently isn't any medication for me, as my doctors repeatedly tell me, "You're doing such a great job handling him," or "Look how far you've come with him." Swirling in my long period of postpartum depression, I feel I've miserably failed with him even when others tell me what an excellent job I have done. A pat on the back doesn't relieve my agony or erase his disorder. How can I let people know that at times I feel ashamed of him? Horribly, I've even thought about how life would have been if he hadn't been born. When he was initially diagnosed, little information about Asperger's syndrome existed, and treatment programs weren't available. Today everyone seems to know of someone who has been diagnosed with some form of autism. Still, there's no cure and I can't place him into a cryogenic vault until a cure is discovered, though it's crossed my mind. Will I ever make the decision to place him in a group home that tolerates no defiant behavior? Could I live, realizing I gave my son away for a sense of normalcy? His disorder affected my marriage and is one reason for my divorce, but it also made me stronger. I've cried enough to fill several oceans; cried myself to sleep and cried from frustration. But I've laughed over his sometimes amusing antics and prayed for sanity to continue dealing with him.

I guess the prayers have been working. I continue slow steps forward, not knowing where they will lead or what's at the end of the road. Gritting my teeth and dealing with "postpartum depression plus twenty," I count love as my medication because I am my autistic son's caregiver and I love my son with super-mom strength, using my sense of humor as support.

Claire Luna-Pinsker is a retired pediatric nurse, wife and the mother of three adult children who now devotes herself full time to writing fiction, nonfiction, and essays on life. Her publishing credits include *Ebony Blood*, a romantic/horror novelette, *Newsday*, *What's Love*, *Affaire De Coeur*, *Our Journey*, *Manic Mom*, and *Born*, and she has been published in *Romantic Hearts*, *True Story*, *Poor Katy's Kab*, and *Chicken Soup For The Caregiver's Soul*, among others.

A Mother's Journal
Susan Norton

September 8, 1983

What's happening to our family? Once, joyful giggles tripped over themselves, and togetherness was something to look forward to as we rushed through our lives. Now, on those rare occasions when we eat together, my stomach churns at the air of rebellion, the cold words, the bloodshot glares, the nasty remarks shot back and forth across the table in staccato time. My protestations are shackled by dread, aimed at a son I no longer know. I wonder, do other parents go through such things? Is this just a stage of growing up? Don't all kids rebel, experiment and then go on with life?

October 3, 1983

I pace the floor, a Bible shaking between my hands, a clutching Christian robed in apprehension, unable to read, the pages blurred by fear, unable to pray, able only to whisper the words, "Help us." Someone once said God has a special regard for the prayers of mothers. Why can't He hear mine? Helpless and hopeless, I wish that someone, somewhere, would heed my silent screams.

October 15, 1983

I slink into my car, cocooned within, feeling safe and sane for a few guarded moments. The sounds of Bach relax my muscles:

tight, twisted, unyielding. Suddenly, the tiniest feeling of joy creeps into my brittle heart. It startles me. Even fleeting happiness scares me so. It makes the despair of my reality seem that much harder to go back to. Instead, I choose to walk around on eggshells, waiting for the next emergency of motherhood, the next challenge to my coping skills. I consciously push that flutter of pleasure aside and resolve instead to opt for a shroud of numbness.

November 11, 1983

I hear a siren in the night. My heart stops. The sound of a helicopter nearby makes my breathing freeze. The telephone rings, my stomach clinches. I stand another solemn vigil through a long and solitary night, once more waiting for the child I used to know, afraid to ask for miracles, praying only for his safe return.

November 23, 1983

Who is this boy? I do not recognize the anger that spits from his mouth, the lifeless, empty stares glued on the face of this stranger. Those beguiling blue eyes that once laughed and charmed me so have gone dead. The mouth that once smiled has gone slack. Yet I know, as only a mother knows, that someplace inside this shell before me, my son still lives.

December 10, 1983

Should I search his room? Does he deserve the privacy to destroy himself? I'm afraid what I will find: liquor bottles, rolling papers, razor blades, mirrors, strange looking glass pipes. What do I do then? I think I'll simply close his door, turn away and pray a little harder. Perhaps, perhaps it will all go away.

December 21, 1983

'Tis the holiday season. I stand at cocktail parties, sipping soda water with lemon, my gaze lost in the glass, wondering about this hold of absolute evil upon my son. I smile sweetly at other mothers, as if my only worries are my son's college choices. Yet, while others stew and fret about their child's SAT scores, I silently pray that mine will simply survive this very night.

January 7, 1984

I am at lunch with girlfriends, daring to enjoy myself. The police call. They are holding him. He's on beer and Quaaludes. "Come and get him," they say. I bolt to my car, tears dripping down my cheeks. I do not bother to stem their flow. I keep repeating, "I don't care." It's not the truth, but somehow I need this mantra to keep my shell of a life from shattering completely. I am clueless as to what to do. From the police station, I take him directly to another psychologist, who says he must be getting mixed up with a bad crowd. "I've learned my lesson this time," my son says. There's a tear in his voice. I have to believe him, for my own sanity.

January 14, 1984

Waiting for the other shoe to drop while wearing vigilance like a cloak. That's how I spend my days and nights. If I give up my son is doomed, lost to a world of darkness. All I know is that I must keep trying to find the single word or phrase that could possibly penetrate his excuses, open him up, free his mind, his heart, his conscience. I'm not above intimidating, buying him off, humbling myself before the angels. It is my job as a mother to fix his world and see him smile again.

February 2, 1984

Where is he? He left so many hours ago. Running interference for him, shielding him from consequences, school officials and police-men has become my full-time job. I pay him to read drug pam-phlets. I beg. I bribe. I threaten. After each disaster, I know he must have learned his lesson this time. But I'm not learning mine. I drive by his school to see if his car is there. I creep over to it and check the trunk for signs of illegal drugs. His life is measured in six packs, dime bags and grams. So is mine. The merry-go-round continues. Neither of us can get off.

May 5, 1984

This date is branded in my memory: the day he is hospitalized. I trick him by saying that he is only going to meet with another professional and then go on to school. I will never forget the sight of him stepping through those metal doors. They slammed with such finality; it sliced my heart open. I knew at that moment that he would never forgive me. I might have lost my son, but just maybe he will live to find and save himself. I question the intake counselor whether he really belongs here. He pats my hand and says, "I asked your son what he would say if I put some bottles of booze, a gram of coke and a baggie of grass before him on this table." He said, "I'd think I'd have died and gone to Heaven." I sign commitment papers with a hand that quivers, feeling drenched in fear and failure.

Professionals calmly speak of his addictions. Don't they know that he's my son? He's barely seventeen. He wears Polo shirts and designer jeans, has short hair, goes to dance class. My mother's heart cries out, "Not my child!" But my adult's mind acknowledges: it is so. The diagnosis plunges forward like a tidal wave: "Middle stages of alcoholism and drug dependency," they tell me. "He's headed on a dead-end course for disaster, and it's killing him." And it's killing me. Dear Lord, it hurts so very much! How can one so young conquer such a foe, spend a life without the chemicals that have become his best friends? I am tethered to pain, unable to escape, incapable of throwing it off. But how much heavier his must be.

I lock his bedroom door when I get home, unable to face the emptiness in both home and heart.

June 7, 1984

My son sits across from me, his foot tapping in beat to the butter-flies in my stomach, and takes my hands in his.

"Get me out of here, Mom. With your help and God's help, I promise I will never use again." His eyes mist. His hands tighten, ever so slightly. His mouth turns up in the most innocent of smiles. He knows that the mention of God is like a rush of fresh air through my resolve. The professionals have warned me that "if his mouth is moving, he is lying." I want nothing more than to take him home, pretend this is not happening, and love him back to normalcy. But my well has run dead dry. "You have to stay," is all I can get past my lips. He surges to his feet. His fists are tight knots, drumming against his thighs, his eyes cold as stones as he slashes past me. I know cold fear.

June 16, 1984

On my first night at the hospital's parents' group, my voice quivers. "Don't try to say it's not my fault. Every cell in my body tells me it is." The rest of the evening I sit, hands buried in my pockets, mouth frozen shut. What a long road lies ahead. Recovery for both of us seems like such an impossible word. Old as it is, it seems like the journey has just begun. So many feelings come up. Why was I so blind to all the signs, so gullible, trusting, defensive, such a failure as a mom? Could I not have looked past his fierce demeanor, the bloodshot eyes, and seen instead the pleadings from those same eyes, his voiceless cries for help?

July 30, 1984

He's coming home, back to his reality as an alcoholic/addict in a swanky suburb of Los Angeles where the roads are paved with denial. What will happen? I only know that I can do nothing but enforce the rules of a contract we have hammered out between us under the direction of the drug program personnel. It may not keep him "clean" but it will keep me sane.

August 5, 1984

Where once a bottle opener hung, sobriety chips now dangle from his key chain: thirty, sixty, ninety days. One step at a time, like an infant learning to walk, he is learning to live.

August 10, 1984

They call it the Family Disease. They tell me I must let him go, cut the cord of maternal enabling, release him to his own future, whatever that may be, step away and no longer rescue him from himself. Trust is like a double-edged sword. I laugh to myself at the word. Like I would ever be able to believe him again? But slowly, tiny step after tiny step, he proves to himself and to me that he can be trusted, and hope makes its home in my heart.

August 27, 1984

Stories tumble from him. He tells me when he was first in rehab, he tried to cut his hand with a sharp piece of metal. He thought that if he hurt himself bad enough, they would have to get him into the regular hospital from which he could easily escape. What got his attention was the reality that he could not feel the slash of sharp metal against his skin. His hand was numb, a reaction to the drugs. It scared him and he thought, "Just maybe, I had better stick around and give this recovery thing a try."

October 19, 1984

Our language changes slowly. Words like "sober" and "clean" become buzzwords and mini-prayers. Slogans clutter our refrigerator door: Easy Does It. Turn It Over. Keep It Simple. Live One Day at a Time, they tell us. What a simple slogan. It rolls off the tongue so easily, slips like ice cream down your throat, but is so hard to do. Like a muscle is built up by exercise, the more we live this day alone, the easier it becomes.

November 28, 1984

Other grieving parents call, voices low and scratched with tears, their stories much the same as mine. I share experiences with them. Desire to help has replaced my pride. They know they are no longer alone. They have found a fellow passenger down a road, a road that is booby trapped by their children's addictions.

December 15, 1984

Kids, trapped by their abuses, come knocking on our door. They are welcomed into our lives. We see past their vacant glares, the litanies of excuses, the rosters of people they blame, their foul, belligerent mouths, and we simply love them until they can love themselves.

March 6, 1985

The past no longer plagues my waking hours. Nightmares are replaced with dreams. Future fears are dimming. Still, I know there is hope, not promise, in this day only.

May 5, 1985

He's one year sober today! He has his future back and so do I. Trust has slowly been rebuilt, brick by brick, kept promise by kept promise. He puts one foot before the other, following a yellow brick road towards tomorrow. Some days he skips, other days his path becomes steep with challenges. But overall, his destiny is of his own design. His life is in his hands, no longer mine.

May 5, 2006

Twenty-two years of sobriety. He has graduated from college, gotten a master's degree, has a job he enjoys and a family he adores. Like all of us, he's gone through the ups and downs of life, traveled highways that twisted and turned, some to dead ends, others to beyond the sun. The journey continues.

Published in over 70 literary journals, magazines, anthologies, newspapers, on greeting cards, in two art exhibits, a cruise brochure, a tear-off calendar, and even fortune cookies, Susan Norton has received ten awards for her writing. With her writing partner, she has published a seven-book series entitled *Pyramid Pal's Adventures in Eating*. Her latest adventure is her foray into the world of travel writing.

(continued from page 137)

Paying for Hospice

Hospice is paid for through the Medicare Hospice Benefit, the Medicaid Hospice Benefit, and most private insurers. If a person does not have coverage through Medicare, Medicaid, or a private insurance company, hospice will work with the person and their family to ensure needed services can be provided.

More than 90% of hospices in the United States are certified by Medicare. Eighty percent of people who use hospice care are over the age of 65 and are thus entitled to the services offered by the Medicare Hospice Benefit. This benefit covers virtually all aspects of hospice care with little out-of-pocket expense to the person or family. In addition, most private health plans and Medicaid in 48 states (Connecticut, New Hampshire, and Puerto Rico excepted) and the District of Columbia cover hospice services.

Sometimes a person's health improves or her illness goes into remission. If that happens, the patient's doctor may feel that the patient no longer needs hospice care. Also, the patient always has the right to stop getting hospice care, at any time, for any reason. If she chooses to stop hospice care, she will receive the type of Medicare coverage that she had before electing hospice. If one is eligible, one can go back to hospice care at any time.

What Does Medicare Cover Under Hospice?

Medicare defines a set of hospice *core services*, which means that hospices are required to provide this set of services to each person they serve, regardless of the person's insurance. Medicare covers and pays for nearly all of the costs of the following services:

- Doctor services

- Nursing care (usually once a week)

- Medical equipment (like wheelchairs, walkers, hospital beds, oxygen)

- Medical supplies (like bandages and catheters)

- Medications for symptom control and pain relief

- Short-term care in the hospital, including respite and inpatient for pain and symptom management

- Home health aide and homemaker services, if desired by the patient

- Physical and occupational therapy as appropriate

- Speech therapy as appropriate

- Social work services

- Dietary counseling

- Grief support to help the patient and family

The patient will only have to pay part of the cost for outpatient medications and inpatient respite care.

What Is Not Covered by the Medicare Hospice Benefit

- *Treatment intended to cure your illness.* The patient will receive comfort care to help manage symptoms related to the illness for which the patient was admitted to hospice. Comfort care includes medications for symptom control and pain relief, physical care, counseling, and other hospice services. Under the hospice benefit, Medicare will not pay for treatment where the goal is to cure the illness. One should talk with one's doctor if the doctor is thinking about potential treatment to cure the illness, and discuss this issue with hospice. A patient always has the right to stop getting hospice care and receive the "traditional" Medicare coverage he had before electing hospice.

- *Medications not directly related to the patient's hospice diagnosis.* The hospice uses medicine, equipment, and supplies to optimize the patient's quality of life. Hospice team members will consult with the hospice physician and will inform the patient and the family which medications are covered and which ones are not covered under the Medicare Hospice Benefit. Medications to treat the patient's other unrelated medical conditions will continue to be paid for by his regular medication plan.

- *Care from another provider that is providing the same care that the patient is getting from hospice.* All care that a hospice patient receives for his illness must be given by his hospice team. A patient can continue to see other physicians for other medical conditions not related to his hospice diagnosis.

- *Nursing home room and board.* The patient may receive hospice services wherever he lives, even in a nursing home; however, the Medicare Hospice Benefit does not pay for nursing home room and board.

(continued on page 168)

The Reward

Rosemary Banks

"Go-to-skoo."

My son is twisting his lips like he is trying to kiss the ceiling. I turn away from brown arms and eyes that beg me to say the words back.

But I'm not going there with Diop this morning.

I see my autistic son, his gaze a convoluted mix of ebullience and panic.

After giving birth to Diop and his twin sister, Nzinga, I believed that unconditional love would follow like breast milk. But instead our lives became a series of trials through which I learned that until you are confronted with severely life-changing situations, you can never know the extent of your capacity to love.

Here his little happy-ass is again; laying an inch-square picture of a yellow school bus on his shirt on the ironing board. I raise the steaming iron to avoid burning it. We've been through it so many times before.

"Come on, D, the bus will be here in a minute."

He holds up the picture. "Go-to-skoo." I pretend to ignore him. He is garrulous with PECS, the acronym for Picture Exchange

Communication System. PECS is supposed to be especially helpful for children with autism who struggle to articulate almost everything, like my son. But Diop is mostly working my nerves with it.

"Go. To. Skoo," Diop says, again.

"You're gonna get burned, Buddy."

I place the iron on the washing machine so it will not fall off the ironing board, which he will bump as he stomps into the next room, shouting, "Football on Fox, football on Fox." Diop remembers catchy phrases from television or radio, or something somebody said, and uses them as his own private word stock—totally out of context.

I'm rushing. Trying to iron another shirt for him to wear to school this morning because the one I laid out last night is too small. The Risperdal the neurologist prescribed for three years to help his hyperactivity caused him to gain a couple of pounds each month. Now he's nearly one hundred and fifty pounds. Thank God, at eight years old he's already five feet.

The fact that I'm getting him ready to go to school means nothing to Diop; he needs to hear me say it. Which I would've been happy to do if that would end it. But in seconds he'll be back in my face asking me to repeat, "Go to school." It is so irritating I can't take it. So, I give in.

Today is Saturday morning. Nzinga is watching cartoons and Diop is playing Nintendo, turning it on and off to hear the theme music. I'm reading in bed. Nzinga runs in, drops the mail on the bed, and runs back to her cartoon. Among the bills is a formal-looking letter from Diop's school for children with developmental disabilities. *What now?* I think as I tear open the letter.

"Congratulations," it reads, "Diop Banks has been chosen student of the year."

I'm immediately pissed. How fucking patronizing can they be at this school? He takes up a sheet of paper to write his four-letter name, and he's student of the year? Come on. But what really pisses me off is the ceremony next Saturday afternoon. How is Diop going to sit through an awards ceremony?

Lately, it seems I'm always on some level of profound irritability. Deep down I am still angry at God and the world about who my son turned out to be. I breathe, deeply, put on some semblance of a happy face and go tell Diop. "Guess what, Mr. D, you've been chosen student of the year at your school." I hug him.

He pushes me back and says with urgency, "McDonald's, please."

I roll my eyes. "No McDonald's for breakfast. Nice try."

I promised Nzinga we'd go to the movies today because I didn't take them last week for one reason or another. It's probably best that we don't go anywhere today, either; Diop has been having bowel movement accidents the whole week, at school and at home. I was disgusted. He'd worn pampers until he was five, special big hospital green ones from a medical supply company. Even now I wipe him after each BM.

Going to see movies has become a brand-new exciting option for us—one of the public places we can now go like regular people without Diop acting inappropriately. Diop is obsessed with necks. To touch or stare at one intently is a thrill for him. He'll walk up to strangers and try to touch their necks, so I always hold his hand. At the theater, Diop will sit somewhat still and quiet as long as we have popcorn and drinks. After that he starts shouting out embarrassing things like, "Wheel of Fortune, Pat Sajak, ginger-bread, cheeseburger, New Mexico."

We're watching a kids' movie, *Juwanna Man*, which Nzinga thought Diop might like because it's a comedy about a basketball team. Everything is going okay. Diop is whispering, "cheeseburger, gingerbread." We're laughing. Then we hear Diop grunt. *Please God, let him just be clearing his throat.* I hold my breath, keep my eyes on the screen, but I'm listening intently for Diop. I hear the grunt again. The reflection of the screen flickers across the pained faces of Nzinga and me. It's as though we're in a movie, and watching one.

"Deee-op," Nzinga scolds.

What to do now? Should I take him to the women's bathroom and try to clean him up with people staring at us? And how could I clean him? Take off his soiled underwear and throw it in the wastebasket and return him to the theater with Diop wearing no underpants?

I look at Nzinga, sitting dejected with her shoulders hunched, her little brown hands folded. To have twins so completely different is a blessing and a curse. I will never give either what they need. "Fuck it, watch the movie." I sit back.

"Mom, don't say that word."

"I said *love it*, watch the movie."

Diop grunts again. I look at my son. His handsome face scrunched, eyes almost shut to little slits. His hands grip the arms of his seat. He pushes, and finally sighs. Desperation washes over me like a hot flash. I think of how much easier my life would be without this fat young boy with curly black hair and dimples. *My life wasn't supposed to be like this.*

For the Student of the Year ceremony I decide to get Diop a suit and tie, or a dashiki and matching kufi, but as always things do not go according to plan. Divorce and single parenting were followed by poverty. While I'm trying to shop for these things at Deptford Mall, the car breaks down like it does every month. I turn the key to shut off the motor but the key comes out and the motor stays on—there goes the money for something special for Diop.

The Saturday of the awards ceremony has arrived too fast. At least Diop's BM problems have been resolved. His new medication was the problem, and once we abandoned it the daily accidents stopped as well. Now I'm thankful to only wipe him after the standard BM.

The car is good to go, even though smoke from burning oil billows out the tailpipe like some abominable genie, and it loses power if I try to go over forty miles an hour. "Look at the huge puffy white clouds, Mom," Nzinga points at a brilliant sky. I had forgotten the sky, trees, flowers—that it was spring melding into summer. "Yeah, girl," I smile back, thankful she is oblivious to our wretchedness. Diop stops sucking his thumb and jumps into the conversation, "Pat Sajak." Nzinga and I burst out laughing, we know what Diop will say next and we say it with him with exact intonations. "And Van-na White." Diop grins and rocks back and forth. For this moment, away from public gaze, I love my children madly—we are a family.

We find a seat in the midst of faculty and aides from Diop's school. I didn't realize this was a regional event and that Diop's school had selected him as their representative. Diop starts squirming almost immediately. One of the aides gives him a Star Wars book. His teacher Ellen is one of the best he's had since he started school at two and a half. She is a pale, slim, middle-aged woman—intelligent, confident and unassuming. I can see that dignity is the intent as each child is introduced by the emcee. Diop is lying on the floor, kicking the chair to hear the metal vibration and humming loudly. One of the aides takes him for a walk.

With Diop gone I pay closer attention to the program. I'm distinctly aware of the open show of feelings from the children. There are no defenses among them, which is what we all fear as parents—their vulnerability—yet, it's so damn refreshing not to hear blasé, clever comments of cynicism and sarcasm.

A young boy steps forward, throws his arms up and shouts into the microphone in the dialect typical of Down's, "I am the greatest," like Ali. Without thinking, I'm starting to smile. What a great spirit he has. I'm startled to find myself actually feeling the joy and pride these children are showing, as though some small window of vulnerability from my past has been jarred open without my intent. I start to clap harder, proud for each kid.

A young girl with curly black hair and green eyes approaches the microphone with her mother; her father stands behind, intense, wearing a yarmulke. She pauses before talking, as she looks at the audience, the same way we are all looking at her. I can't help thinking to myself that a normal person would not have dared stand in front of an audience and take the time to acknowledge our faces. We with so-called intelligence try to efficiently whiz through most every event in our lives.

The girl smiles into the microphone, and as our audience anticipation peaks she breathes, "Wow." When she adds nothing to it, we clap out of politeness, but also from *wanting* to understand.

Diop is back and almost immediately they call his name. "Our student of the year from Gloucester County Special Services is Diop Molefi Banks. Diop is an African name meaning 'scholar.' He loves school. Everyone hopes that someday Diop will learn how to play the drums—so he'll stop beating on the desk. Ladies and gentlemen, Diop Banks."

We go to the front of the auditorium with Diop walking his boyish, gangling strut (the way comedians do when they imitate retarded people) between his teacher and me with Nzinga on my other side. Diop starts clapping. Clapping is one of my son's favorite pastimes: he wakes in the morning applauding sunrise. Unexpectedly for Diop, the audience claps with him. He is baffled that unlike Nzinga and Mommy, who tell him to shut up already, people have actually joined him.

I say to the audience, "Diop thanks you and Nzinga and I thank you so much," and step back. Holding Diop and Nzinga's hands before them, my spirit feels awakened and uplifted.

Rosemary Banks was awarded a master's degree in creative writing from Rosemont College and in liberal studies from Rutgers University. Her short story, *Being Zarathustra*, has been nominated for publication in *Best American Voices of 2009*.

(continued from page 160)

How Are Palliative Care and Hospice Healthcare Professionals Different?

Caring for dying patients and for those who suffer from chronic and severe illnesses with uncertain prognoses requires specialized training, experience with an interdisciplinary approach, and specific clinical skills. In particular, the clinician who provides hospice and palliative care must be competent in clinical communication, management of symptoms (physical, emotional, and psychological), working in interdisciplinary teams, and planning for continuity of care.

Why Good Communication Is Important

The ability to communicate well with both patient and family is paramount in palliative care. In the beginning, it enables the physician to deliver bad news in a compassionate and supportive way, assess the patient's and the family's knowledge and understanding of the disease process, determine the factors that they consider important to the quality of life, and discuss goals and preferences for future care. For physicians who do not have this training or these skills, communication about a serious diagnosis may be traumatic, awkward, or sometimes nonexistent. As the illness progresses, regular communication about the course of illness and the patient's needs and expectations enables the healthcare team to provide the most appropriate care for the patient and support for the family. A common example is where the patient has longstanding diabetes, heart disease, chronic kidney failure, emphysema, and now is minimally conscious and suffering respiratory failure requiring long-term support with a breathing machine. Healthcare providers not trained in palliative care may ask the family,

"Do you want us to do everything for your loved one?" A question like this is not productive as it does not assess the family's understanding of the situation nor the patient's goals of care, but does generate feelings of guilt and helplessness.

Communication continues to be important after the patient's death, because the period of bereavement poses major challenges and increased risks of medical and psychiatric illness for family members.

Patients whose cultural background and language differ from that of the physician present special challenges and rewards and need to be approached in a culturally sensitive manner (more on this later on). Physicians also need to communicate effectively with colleagues and interdisciplinary team members to achieve the best care for their patients.

Why Good Symptom Management Is Important

For clinicians not trained in palliative care and hospice, pain and other distressing symptoms are used to diagnose illnesses, but are seldom treated in and of themselves to make the patient feel better. Symptom management in palliative care and hospice includes not only the assessment and treatment of physical symptoms but emotional and psychological symptoms as well. Physical symptoms that can contribute to discomfort, disability, and dependence include pain, difficulty breathing, constipation, nausea and vomiting, confusion, fatigue, and poor appetite. Emotional and psychological symptoms include depression, anxiety, confusion, cognitive impairment, fear and agitation or sedation, as well as spiritual and existential angst.

Pain is the most common symptom of terminal illness, reported by 84% of patients with cancer and 67% of patients dying of other causes. Other common symptoms reported by dying patients include trouble with breathing (49%), nausea and vomiting (33%), sleeplessness (40%), depression (36%), loss of appetite (47%), and constipation (36%). Other symptoms that become more prevalent with increasing age include mental confusion, loss of bladder and bowel control, difficulty seeing and hearing, and dizziness.

At present, the identification and management of many symptoms, including pain, remain less than what could be hoped for. Under-treatment of symptoms is common in elderly patients whether they have cancer or other chronic conditions, whether they reside in long-term care settings (45% to 80% prevalence) or in the community, and whether they are white or are members of minority groups. Under-treatment of pain in the elderly may be more common in patients who are women, are members of minority groups, or have mild to moderate cognitive impairment. Clinicians may contribute to under-treatment of pain through lack of proper pain assessment procedures, fear of prescribing opioid medications, misconceptions regarding both the efficacy of nonpharmacologic pain management strategies, attitudes of the elderly toward such treatments, and legitimate concerns about drug interactions and side effects. Poorly controlled pain can lead to depression, social withdrawal, and a diminished quality of life in patients who already might not have a long time to live. Good assessment and treatment of pain and other symptoms require a two-way collaboration between the clinician and the patient or caregiver. Educating and involving the patient and family as partners in care are key to the successful management of symptoms.

Why It Is Important to Work in Interdisciplinary Teams
When a person is seriously ill or dying, no single discipline or specialty is able to manage all the domains in which that

person may be suffering and needs help. Each discipline has its expertise and must know enough about the strengths of other disciplines to know when to call for help. Over the years, I have encountered many situations where a team approach works best. Some examples follow:

Christine, a young woman dying of widely spread colon cancer, is deeply religious, but is now in a spiritual crisis because she cannot make sense of why she is dying an untimely death. She refuses to take any medications and prays for salvation. As the doctor, I tried to simplify her medications as much as possible to keep her symptoms at bay, but our pastoral care chaplain was much more able to meet her needs.

Mr. and Mrs. Smith, both 85 years old, are chronically ill and need help with their daily activities. They need to privately hire aides to help them, but are short on cash. They did have a second house and our social worker was able to give them information about obtaining a reverse mortgage so they could pay for the aides.

Jack was a 50-year-old man with severe diabetes, chronically high blood sugars, and related wounds. I was able to prescribe an insulin and wound care regimen but I needed my nursing colleagues to teach him how to accurately check his sugars and care for his wounds, and my nutritionist colleagues to advise him of appropriate dietary choices.

Why Planning for Continuity of Care Is Important

For a clinician not trained in hospice/palliative care, his scope of practice tends to focus on the location of care, whether it is the emergency room, hospital, clinic, or nursing home. Hospice and palliative care professionals are trained to think more on a "systems" level, knowing the relationships between each location or type of practice, and ensuring that information flows from one location to another in order to keep continuity of care.

Hospice provides 24/7 access to on-call nurses and doctors who can respond to acute symptoms at night or during weekends, thereby avoiding unnecessary visits to the emergency department. Grief and bereavement support is another aspect of continuity of care. If a person dies in a hospital or nursing home, the intense working relationships between the family and the health care team dissolves virtually overnight. But with hospice, there is built-in bereavement follow-up and counseling to ensure that the family or caregiver is not forgotten.

(continued on page 193)

Needed

B. Lynn Goodwin

"When are you planning on going to the grocery store?" my mother asked after our trip to the hairdresser followed by a late lunch at Emil Villa's. I'd taken her back to her condo, helped her open her mail, and I thought my day was over.

"I'll go right now."

"Don't go now. You don't have time." I did though, and we both knew it. I hated being reminded that I had no life.

"When would you like me to go, Missus?" I asked with all the patience I could muster. She was Missus and I was Person, names that kept us unique and reminded us that we loved each other, even in trying times.

"I don't care." Fists clenched, she shook her arms for emphasis. "Go tomorrow or the next day or whenever you want to."

We did this dance every day. She needed help; I needed space. She feared I would abandon her, while I feared that her blood pressure would soar, causing another stroke.

It would be four years before I knew that a disease was eating her brain, robbing her of logical thought, and returning her to the emotional dependence of a child. I had no idea I was engaged in a psychological battle with a woman who was losing her ability to think logically.

I put on my patient face and said, "I've got time and I want to go now. What would you like me to bring?"

She looked up with vacant, pleading eyes. Four years later I would call them Alzheimer eyes. "Can we look at the list?"

"Sure." She'd spent all one afternoon sitting at a wobbly card table typing the list, letter by letter, then going back and X-ing out her mistakes. I offered to type on either her typewriter or my computer while she dictated, but she said, "I have to do something for myself." Watching her struggle with the scraps of memory lurking in her brain made me want to scream. I dug my fingernails into my crossed arms until little red half-moons dotted my elbows.

I found the typed grocery list in a stack of old Saks catalogues. "Would you like Lean Cuisines Chicken Chow Mein or Chicken with Vegetables?"

"Don't bring me that thing you brought last time. It only had one piece of meat and it was all fat."

Beef Portobello was the culprit. Furious and frustrated, she'd waved the fatty piece of meat on the end of her fork, then slammed the half-empty plastic tray on the counter. "Don't ever bring me this again!"

Like I have X-ray vision. Like I use it to check the contents of every box, and deliberately thwart your food life by bringing you only substandard packages. I breathed deeply. "Why don't I see what's in the freezer?"

In my best Vanna White imitation, I pulled out each item, turned, showed it, and called out its name. If I read the names while I looked in the freezer, she couldn't hear me. This was simpler. Besides my Vanna poses were entertaining, and I loved my mother's approval, though at 48 I should have been far too old to care.

"Take some money out of the dresser." I did as I was told though I already had her money in her section of our wallet. Nothing was exclusively mine anymore.

Crisp fall air filled my lungs as I scurried to my car. I looked up at the bare spots already showing on the trees. I didn't know yet that Alzheimer's speckled her brain with holes in exactly the same way as fallen leaves made holes in the trees. I wondered if this was the last year she would see the leaves turn.

If I had known about her disease, maybe I could have stopped trying to be the perfect daughter. Maybe I could have loved her for needing me instead of craving her approval. Maybe I could have recognized that I was an adult daughter, doing what needed to be done.

I realize now that her behavior contradicted everything I knew about Alzheimer's. She didn't wander around undressed or leave the stove on. She was just being herself—only more so.

When I came back from the store, she thanked me profusely. "I don't know what I would do without you, Person."

"No problem." My resentment disappeared whenever we were apart.

"Did you get everything on the list?"

"They didn't have those cookies you like, but I found everything else."

"When will they?

I stared for a moment. "They don't make them anymore, remember, Missus?"

"Nobody ever makes anything I like."

B. Lynn Goodwin's work has been published in *Hip Mama, The Oakland Tribune, The Contra Costa Times, The Danville Weekly, Staying Sane When You're Dieting, Small Press Review, Dramatics*

Magazine and numerous e-zines. She edits and writes reviews and author interviews for *Writer Advice*, www.writeradvice.com. Information about her book, *You Want Me To Do What?—Journaling for Caregivers* and about journaling workshops conducted by e-mail may be found on the website.

Love Lessons
Laura Shumaker

It was February 16th; two days after the Valentine's Day storm paralyzed the Northeast. I had just finished my continental breakfast—a rubbery muffin and weak coffee—at a mediocre hotel near the Philadelphia Airport. My flight from Oakland had arrived late the night before, following hours of delays, and I was tired and jittery. I was on my way to pick up my twenty-year-old son, Matthew, who is autistic, at his special school in rural Pennsylvania. He had been begging me to take him to Washington D.C. since he'd enrolled at the school three years before, and I thought it would be fun to go over the President's Day weekend break.

When the storm hit I almost backed out, but maternal love and guilt pushed me forward. Sending Matthew to a residential school was the last thing that my husband and I thought we would ever do. But it was absolutely necessary.

Matthew always wanted to be something he can't be: a regular guy like his two younger brothers. In fact, Matthew didn't just want to be a regular guy, but *the* guy—the poisonous plant and weed expert, and the lawn care authority of our northern California community. He would often be seen at our local hardware store with his large hands wrapped around a bottle of weed killer, studying the label intently. My socially awkward son would approach strangers with warnings about deadly nightshade, oleander and water hemlock. Some would snicker and walk away.

Just a few days into his 16th year, Matthew decided that he should drive a car like a regular guy, and drove my car through a wall in our garage. There were other close calls. During his freshman year at high school, he observed a guy pushing his girlfriend flirtatiously and then tapping her on the head. When Matthew tried the same move with too much force, I was summoned to his school to find him crying in the principal's office. "Joe did it to Sue, and she liked it!"

Just when we thought things were calming down following that incident, a letter arrived from an attorney asking us to contact him about a bicycle accident involving Matthew. Matthew had collided with a young boy on his bike the month before.

"Matthew," I asked him, "what's this about a bike accident?"

"Who told you?"

"Someone sent me a letter. Was the boy you bumped into hurt?"

"Pretty much"

Dear God.

"Was he bleeding?"

"Probably. Am I in trouble?"

It became clear that Matthew was no longer safe in the community where he had grown up, and his impulsive actions were putting others in peril. He needed more supervision, more than we or the local school could provide. So we searched for the ideal facility for him, and found this one in Pennsylvania.

My other son's words played in my head as I approached Matthew's home. "Matthew would be really good looking if he wasn't autistic." As unkind as it sounded, it was true, and still is. Matthew is very handsome, with a tall and solid frame, broad shoulders, and sandy blonde hair. His eyebrows arch dramatically to frame his brown eyes, and his jaw is square and masculine. But his exaggerated expressions and awkward body carriage make him stand out in a crowd. His forehead twists with intensity, he smiles too suddenly and his hungry-for-friendship gaze is desperate. And he insists on trimming his own bangs, with unfortunate results.

When I arrived at the home, Matthew was waiting on the porch. He smiled widely as I pulled into the snowy driveway of the house he shared with two other students and his house parents, Dawn and Lazlo. That old familiar lump made its way back to my throat. It was clear that he had just cut his bangs again, another botched job. He was wearing jeans, black snow boots and a thin T-shirt, even though it was only 28 degrees. He was blowing the snow with the leaf blower that I'd given him for Christmas.

"He's been so excited about this trip," Dawn said as she loaded Matthew's bag in the car. Matthew had been unusually aggressive about making contact with "hot" girls when his school group went on outings, using suave pickup lines such as "Can I touch your hair?" and "When was the last time you had a seizure?" When counselors from the school tried to offer suggestions of more appropriate exchanges, Matthew yelled, "Stay out of my business!" The pretty girls had scattered, rolling their eyes, and leaving Matthew angry and inconsolable. I applauded anyone who tried to crack Matthew's socially awkward behavior, but I was losing hope that Matthew would ever be able to enjoy the relationship that he craved.

The drive from Pennsylvania to Washington was stressful as I swerved to avoid shards of ice, remnants of the storm, that flew off cars, trucks and tree limbs. Matthew seemed oblivious to my angst, and played Beatles music loudly, replaying the first thirty seconds of *Octopus's Garden* over and over each time we entered a new state. By the time we got to D.C. I was ragged and hungry. While I was thrilled to see the Washington Monument, the White House and the Jefferson Memorial for the first time, I worried that it was all too much for Matthew, who was smiling but flapping his hands and rocking double time. We found a pizza place (Matthew's first meal while traveling must be pizza) and Matthew settled down after eating his cheese pizza "with nineteen French fries on the side" before heading back to our hotel for the night.

During breakfast at our hotel the next morning, I bit my lip as Matthew leered awkwardly at our attractive young waitress while ordering three Belgian waffles and a side order of sausage. "First time in D.C.?" she asked, "You have *got* to go to the Botanical Gardens! Look," she said, pointing at our map, "It's just about six blocks away, right next to the Capitol."

"I'm smart about gardens, I tell you," Matthew said earnestly, trying to impress, "and you should stay away from oleanders. They're poisonous." The waitress rushed away, stifling laughter, leaving me with the heavy feeling in my chest that mothers get when people laugh at their children.

I panicked when I first saw the enormous glass conservatory that housed the botanical gardens and the swarm of people streaming in. Clearly, this was a popular week for middle school tour groups in Washington. A pack of girls in their early teens was bunched in front of us, giggling uncontrollably.

"Those girls are hot!" Matthew said loudly enough to elicit wary looks from the chaperones.

"They're too young to be hot," I shot back nervously as Matthew pushed towards the entrance. "Stay away from them or you'll get in trouble."

"Let me go in first," Matthew said, still eyeing the young teens. "I don't want people to think I came here with my mother."

"That's fine," I said. "But Matthew, this is Washington D.C." I pointed at the pair of armed security guards at the entrance. "It's important that we stay together and use our best manners. Do you understand?"

"If I don't use my manners, will they think I'm a bad guy?" Matthew asked, raising his brows slyly.

"They might. You're a big guy, you know how to behave."

I tried to suppress the sinking feeling that I'd already lost control of the day, that this entire trip had been a bad idea, that the reward for my sacrifice would be heartache for me and frustration for Matthew. It had been easy to fantasize about this trip from California, where the magnificence of Washington was uncluttered by snow, crowds, and hot middle school girls. But here we were, at the entrance of the Botanical Gardens. I had to try to make our day a successful one.

Matthew followed the group of young middle-schoolers past the security guards, darting through a series of automatic sliding doors that separated the collections of plants. He was working so hard to distance himself from me that he looked suspicious, and I looked like an undercover agent tracking him. This was not a good place to be running after an oddly behaving son, and I caught Matthew by the arm just as a security guard started marching toward us.

"Is everything all right here?" he demanded. "My mother keeps following me," wailed Matthew. "I need some space. I want to be independent!"

"Of course you do," said the guard, glancing at the hacked bangs that explained all. "But you need to stay together while you're in this building."

Gripped by his desire to connect with pretty girls, Matthew took off again once the guard turned his back, and I followed until he raced through the exit and turned to me, stomping his foot. "Stop stalking me!" he yelled, echoing the words he'd heard directed toward him so many times before. I felt like the young mother whose child was having a meltdown at the grocery store—if only I could just pick Matthew up and disappear into my minivan. Instead, I had to remain calm.

"I have a great idea," I said, "Let's drive to Virginia! You've never been there before."

"Or we could go there first," Matthew said, pointing to the Capitol Building. There was a line curving around the imposing marble steps, also protected by armed security guards. I took a breath. "Can you promise to stay with me and walk slowly," I implored, "and will you remember that this is the most important place *in the world* to follow the rules?"

Fortunately, the line that led to the entrance of the Capitol was moving quickly. It wasn't until we got to the security checkpoint that I learned we were in the line for the gallery that overlooked the Senate floor. There was a special Saturday session debating the Iraq war. Matthew and I were led into the second of three rows that overlooked the Senate floor, where John Warner was speaking. No walls, no bulletproof glass...just open air and the Senate floor right before us. A camera crew was taping the proceedings for CSPAN. Then I noticed five very good looking college-age girls seated in the row behind us.

God help me...

The hot flashes I'd experienced before were nothing compared to the *whoosh* of heat that rushed through me now. Matthew promptly got down to business, leaning back and flirting loudly and awkwardly with the co-ed behind him. She shook her head and motioned for him to turn around, which he did with a sly smirk.

"Talking is not allowed here," I whispered firmly. "I'm serious."

"OK!" he yelled. I glanced at the security guards. Matthew had gotten their attention. What would they do if he erupted again? Just as Carl Levin rose to speak, Matthew twisted around again, tapped the knee of another girl behind him and waved at her.

"*Cut it out!*" she whispered, then looked at her friends in disbelief. While I was frantically thinking of a way to coax Matthew out peacefully, the girls got up and left in disgust. Matthew rose to leave with them, but one of the security guards motioned for him to stay seated. Matthew looked surprised, hesitated, then sat down and faced forward. His face turned red, and tears poured down his face. Dianne Feinstein made her way to the podium. I looked pleadingly at the security guard, and he came to my aid. "Let's go, son," he said kindly, his arm outstretched, and my sobbing son and I filed out of the gallery.

Once outside in the hallway, Matthew confided to the security guard that he wanted a hot girlfriend because he was healthy. I put my arm around Matthew's shoulder and we left the Capitol. I wondered what I could say about this experience that would make sense to him. The obvious explanation would be that since 9/11, it was more important than ever keep a low profile. But how in the world could I communicate that to a person devoid of common sense?

"Those girls really hurt my feelings," Matthew said as we exited into the cold. "They weren't nice."

"I know, Matthew, but you know what? One time when I was your age, something like this happened to me, too."

"Really? Where were you?"

"Well, I was in church, and some really cool guys were sitting behind me. I decided to talk to them."

"Then what happened?"

"I started to talk to them and they told me to shut up!"

"Then what did you do?"

"I started crying. Then my mother, your grandma, walked me out of the church."

"Was she angry with you?"

"No, she knew that I felt bad because the boys yelled at me. She explained to me that at church, you are not supposed to talk. And the boys knew that and didn't want to get in trouble."

"Oh." Matthew was quiet for about a minute, and wiped his runny nose on the sleeve of his pale blue sweater.

"But Mom," he asked, his voice quavering, "did the boys actually think you were nice?"

"I don't know," I said. "I never saw them again. But later there were other boys who thought I was nice."

"That's good. I'm done talking about the girls now. Can we have lunch in Virginia?"

We headed toward Virginia, and as Matthew cued up *Octopus's Garden* on the car's CD player, it occurred to me that this silly ritual had a purpose: it distracted Matthew's heavy, longing heart. As littered with roadblocks as it was, Matthew's search for a meaningful relationship, his need to be a regular guy, was as important as anyone's.

I looked back wistfully as we drove away from the Washington Monument and Jefferson Memorial that we wouldn't visit.

I'll see them next time.

Laura Shumaker is the author of the forthcoming memoir, A *Regular Guy: Growing Up With Autism* (Landscape Press, 2008), and a regular contributor to *NPR Perspectives*. A columnist for *The Autism Perspective*, her essays have also appeared regularly in the *San Francisco Chronicle*, the *Contra Costa Times*, the *East Bay Monthly* and *Hallmark Magazine*.

Part V
Forgiveness

...of one's self or a loved one frequently grows
from the experience of giving care.

Visitors

M.C. Winters

"Your father and I want to go to Ryan's christening on Sunday."

I hesitated. This would be my first time alone with my grandfather since we'd brought him home to my parents' house from the hospital.

"Look," my mother whispered, so he wouldn't hear. "I don't know what I would have done without you. But I've been stuck in this house for weeks now without a moment to myself or a moment to rest. I've got to get out."

For some time now, I had been "visiting" my parents after work most weekdays and full-time on weekends, trying to lighten my mother's load, trying to lighten my grandfather's pain and disorientation. But it was beginning to look—my grandfather was beginning to look—as if there might not be much time left for visiting. Disease had ruined his body. He had shrunk to a stunningly skeletal eighty pounds; he was too weak to sit unassisted for more than a few minutes; he was in constant pain. As frail as he had become, he was still an ungainly, dangerous burden: with his flailing, scarecrow hands and pointy elbows, he had given my petite, middle-aged mother a black eye as we helped him to the bedside commode. His mind was becoming more and more confused and vague. He had no idea who we were, though he asked for my grandmother, dead now three years, and for my aunt, dead thirty. On good days we rearranged our own lives to care for him, and on bad days we simply put our lives on hold. We were doing everything we could to help him through, to help ourselves through, this sudden set of circumstances for which none of us had been prepared. We were exhausted and bruised, emotionally and physically, from caring for him.

After my parents left for Ryan's christening, my grandfather rested fitfully, wheezing, moaning, calling out unintelligibly to no one in particular—or at least to no one I knew. I sat in the kitchen, writing checks from his account to pay his rent and utilities. He and Ma and I had agreed to this arrangement the afternoon we'd brought him home to the guest room at my parents' house. There'd been no indication, at that time, that he would never recover from his surgery and be unable return to his own apartment and his lifelong independence.

But now, I felt angry and ashamed: despite the entirely good intentions of this logical arrangement, I felt more like a thief with each check I wrote. He'd mostly forgotten our arrangement. He often wondered not only who my mother and father and I were, but also who *he* was, where *here* was, why we *kept* him here, why we were *stealing* his meager funds. I felt angry with myself and him and the medical profession and society and God, and I was angry that I felt ashamed.

I tried to tease him out of his room, to help him to move around a bit, to encourage him to have to something to eat, to remind him that we loved him and he loved us. With great difficulty he sat up and slid his thin, dry feet into his favorite slippers. When he attempted to stand, I came in as if I had just happened to be passing and noticed him there. I smiled and exclaimed, "Hi!" His clothes seemed monstrously large, as if a voracious flannel shirt had tried to eat him but hadn't quite managed to digest his head or fingertips. His face was literally gray. His once lively blue eyes were wide and fearful. He stared at me and then at the floor. I reached toward him, but he pulled back and then swayed to side-step me, careful not to let his arm brush against mine. He walked toward the kitchen, holding onto the wall to keep from tipping, tripping and falling.

I followed him to the kitchen, then reached around to pull out a chair for him. Still looking at the floor, he sat carefully, moaning as his legs bent and his body connected with the cushioned seat. I began chatting about nothing, to continue, for his sake, the pretense that he was just visiting my parents, and that I was just visiting him. To pretend, for my own sake, that I wasn't ashamed to be "caught" writing his checks, or to see him in this condition.

Though exhausted, he appeared restless; though confused, he was angry, too. He spat the words "fuck" and "fucking" at me. If I understood the context then, I don't remember it now. But they fell on me, direct hits to the chest. My lungs collapsed; my head ached; my vision swam; my hearing blurred. I had never heard my grandfather—who had always stood so tall and straight and behaved with such dignity, and who had always cared so much for his family—raise his voice in anger or swear.

My immediate defensive reaction was that this was not *my* grandfather. I was overwhelmed by the evidence that some other consciousness was fighting for control of his body, and by the realization of his inability to recognize it, to fight it, and to banish it—and of our inability to banish it for him. I flushed and sent my grandfather to his room as if he were a child. And then, as if I were a child, I scurried into the bathroom and locked the door.

I listened as he shuffled slowly, carefully, back to his room, suddenly no longer the disconnected and abusive stranger, but merely a defeated child. Upset as I was, I found myself thinking, *I should have helped him. What if he'd fallen?*

Then, softly, barely recognizable as my grandfather's voice: "Maggie?"

He had always called me Maggie. He was the only one I allowed to do so. "Just a minute," I called roughly, reminding us both that *he* was the weak and dependent child, that I was the adult in charge, as if we all did not already know that, as if that fact were not the source of both his and my own confusion and anger.

I was still hot, flushed and terrified that he would swear at me again, or that I would hurt his feelings more than I already had. I was terrified that he would give me a shiner, or that I would accidentally injure his brittle body. I rinsed my face quickly, inhaled, opened the bathroom door and walked into his room.

He lay on the bunched disposable pad on the thin, uncomfortable sofa bed, hands clasped behind his head, staring at the ceiling. He grabbed weakly at my hand, pulled me down to sit on the bed, and looked at me. Lucid! And tearful.

"I'm sorry, Maggie. I really am."

There hadn't been time for me to wonder which was worse—seeing him so angry and hearing him swear, or seeing him so thoroughly beaten by life, by death, and now by me.

Contrite, also tearful: "So am I."

"I just don't understand what's wrong with me," he said, shaking his head.

"You've been a little sick," I offered. "You've had a tough few weeks, so we brought you home to Ma's and Daddy's to visit and rest up."

"Well, yes, now that you mention it, I haven't been feeling quite like myself lately."

I couldn't help but half-smile at his sad understatement. He looked around. "Yes. I'd like to go home now. Ah, but I guess I'm not up to it yet, am I?"

"No. I am so sorry, but not yet."

He nodded. *He did understand.*

For weeks I'd been hoping for just this chance to connect with him, and I hugged him tentatively. He tried to arrange his arms to hug me.

"Pop, I want to tell you something, and I don't want you ever to forget. You've made Ma's life and Daddy's life and my life and a lot of other people's lives better. I love you, and I'll miss you."

He seemed to consider my words. Still, for all I knew, he could have been wishing for a cigarette, or considering the leaves on the tree outside the window, or envisioning his long-dead parents. Then he looked me in the eye.

"I love you all, too, and I really do hope I've helped you all along your paths."

He lay back, looked at the ceiling again, and asked me to stay, to hold his hand.

My parents returned home a short time later.

"He didn't eat, but he's sleeping now."

"That's good," they said, though we all knew it was a mixed blessing. We were happy for his temporary respite from pain and fear. But his sleeping during the day virtually guaranteed another wakeful night. While my parents tried to sleep, he would chat with childhood friends in Gaelic, sing old songs we'd never heard, and beg to go "home". But he could never specify what "home" was. Ireland, where his parents had been born? New York City, where he'd been born and survived a difficult childhood? The apartment a few miles from here? Heaven? If my parents were lucky, he'd fall asleep at dawn.

I never told my mother about my anger and shame, or about Pop's moment of lucidity, or about our conversation. And if she ever had a similar conversation with him, she never told me. But it's unlikely.

Soon after this incident (we could never be sure at exactly what moment), Pop went away for good, though his body, occupied by that strange consciousness, lingered for several days.

We try to take comfort in the fact that we did the best we could with the information and resources we had; we mostly fail, because our best was not nearly good enough for a man who deserved so very, very much. My mother still says she takes comfort, too, from Ryan's life—he's a healthy, intelligent, handsome boy, off to college this year. But although I believe that as an adult human being I should be able to find comfort in the infinite circle of life, I find it only in the infinitely small moment my grandfather and I shared—and in the hope that he found some measure of comfort in it, too.

––––––––––

M.C. Winters is author of two articles about gendered language which appeared in the Society for Technical Communication's *Boston Broadside*, several papers about language and literature, and is a contributor to *Legacies: Fiction, Poetry, Drama.*

(continued from page 172)

Accounting for Cultural Differences

The United States is a culturally heterogeneous country. Culture can broadly include race and ethnicity, as well as country of origin, religion, spirituality, values and beliefs, and profession. Medicine has its culture as well, with its attendant values, beliefs, behaviors, and language. Thus, in some cases, hospice patients may be encountering two unfamiliar cultures: that of the mainstream American culture and that of Western medicine.

Cultural traits may have a far-reaching impact on a patient's views on illness, preferences, and ultimate decision-making. Compared with patients from the mainstream culture (most of whom are whites of European descent), people from other cultural backgrounds may be less willing to discuss their wishes about resuscitation, less likely to forego life-sustaining treatment, less likely to use hospice services, and more reluctant to complete advance directives. Also, decisions on care are more often made by the family than by the patient alone. Although many individual variations exist, some frequently encountered examples of cultural differences include the following:

- Hindus traditionally respect the doctor's medical opinion and may request the physician, rather than a family member, be appointed as health care proxy. They may prefer to die at home, preferably on the floor near the earth. After death, the relatives may want to wash the body themselves and dress it in new clothes. Autopsy is not forbidden but is considered distasteful, and cremation is usual.

- Traditional Chinese (and some other Asian) families usually will ask the clinician not to inform the patient about a terminal diagnosis (especially cancer) for fear that the patient will lose hope and die. In these cultures, the patient ideally will be informed after a period of adjustment. Decision-making is often entrusted to the eldest child, usually a son. Patients may not wish to die at home, considering a hospital death less burdensome for the family. Patients may seek traditional therapies, such as acupuncture and herbal medicine, often in conjunction with Western medical care.

• African Americans may decline participation in research studies, because of their long history of abuse as experimental subjects in research. Because of their history of receiving inappropriate under-treatment, they may continue to request aggressive care, even in terminal illness. Also, religious and spiritual beliefs may play a big part in decision-making.

With patients who do not speak English, it is extremely helpful to have access to a trained interpreter who can provide an objective translation and shift the translation burden from family members. This can prevent awkward and inappropriate situations, such as having to ask a male teenager to interpret for his mother who has cervical cancer. Translators may also be able to provide valuable information about patients' cultural attitudes and expectations.

Although it is important to learn about and respect different cultural practices, it is even more important *not* to stereotype or assume that membership in a group automatically determines preferences. Instead, the goal of the hospice and palliative care team is to treat each patient as an individual.

(continued on page 232)

Letting Go

Elizabeth Van Ingen

I heard the car screech out and the garage door roll shut. I sank into a chair at the kitchen table and hid my face in my hands. Let him stay at the Holiday Inn. He'd be all right. It was only a mile and a half down the road. What could I do anyway? Frankly, I was glad he was gone. Where is the sweet but sad love story, I thought? This is terror, every day. In the stillness of the kitchen, I reminded myself that I was with him because I chose to be.

My husband was sick. After a long struggle with doctors to have my fears about Tony's symptoms taken seriously, at the age of 67 he was diagnosed with probable Alzheimer's disease. The disconnect growing between us was not a marital problem that could be fixed, as one doctor suggested, but the result of the disease, which could not be.

The diagnosis did not bring the closure I had expected, but more ambiguity and an overwhelming sense of abandonment. Where were the directions for the rest of my life? I had followed Tony's lead for forty years, literally around the world. Now I had to make the decisions about our future and he wouldn't be able to help me. He didn't respond to me in the loving way he used to. I was fading from his awareness. I stopped expecting any emotional support from him. If I hadn't, every hour of every day would have been a battle.

"I don't know if I can do this, Hanna," I said to Tony's sister. "I am not the nurse type. I can't stand to see Tony so bewildered and angry and out of control. I feel like I'm walking blindfolded, knee deep in mud. I am just stuck."

Her empathy came through the phone as she listened. Then she said, "You don't have to do it, Liz. You can leave; get someone else to take care of him. There are resources. There are homes," and finally, "Some people even divorce."

For a minute, I couldn't speak. "Oh, Hanna," I cried, "He's my husband...forty years...I love him. I could never leave him." Was that too quick a decision, I thought as I put down the phone?

When Tony snapped off the TV while I was watching a program, I stifled my reaction and told myself it really wasn't important. Peace was more important to me than a battle over things that didn't matter, and now, nothing mattered. When he shoved a newspaper between my nose and the book I was reading, or demanded my attention while I was on the phone, or adjusted the curtains I had just arranged, I smiled and said nothing. It really didn't matter. When we planned to leave at 9 A.M. for the two-and-a-half-hour drive to Des Moines to our daughter's house for Christmas, it didn't really matter that we left at noon and delayed her plans by three hours. She and I learned to make flexible plans. He hadn't participated in Christmas for years. "What's Christmas anyhow? Christmas is for stupid people. Go by yourself," he said, throwing the keys and kicking the door.

As I let my work and my interests lose their meaning for me, our life slowed to a near standstill. I thought of myself as having been in a speeding car going 75 miles an hour down the highway, then coming to the outskirts of a town and slowing to 45, then 35, then 25. Now, 15 miles an hour felt comfortable and I was old. I was 61 and old and stuck. We were slipping into a troubled new world, he and I, and no amount of money, education, past history, common sense or love could keep us out. I looked to his side of the bed where that morning he had sat, holding his head in his hands whispering, "My brain isn't working; my brain just isn't working. I feel like a balloon floating this way and that with no one holding the string."

My heart wept. He was losing his mind and I ached to gain control. I stood up from the kitchen table, turned out a few lights and got myself into bed. I wore my bathrobe and socks in bed; I was shivering. I lay on my back staring into the dimness, wondering if I should call the Holiday Inn to see if he had gotten there. No, leave him alone, I thought. Quit interfering. He had to rely on me and yet my presence constantly reminded him that he was losing his mind. "No, not in that drawer," I'd say, "The top drawer, the top drawer." "You don't want to eat now; we just ate." "Get ready; we're leaving in five minutes." My constant help must drive him crazy.

I knew his storming out of the house was not my fault, but something I did had triggered it. I tried to control everything, but I had slipped up. My whole body ached as I lay there remembering. Tony had come downstairs to where I was working in my office in our basement. His calendar was in his hand. He stretched out on the couch and said, "Next week we have to get our tickets for Europe to see my mother, make arrangements for our trip to Holland. Are you with me on this?"

"Trip to Europe?" I said. "No, not really. I don't know if we can manage that." He leaped off the couch, fists in the air. "You're always double crossing me! I'll go without you! I can find some lady to go with me! You stay here by yourself! I'm going to do what I want!" He charged at me, red faced, finger pointing, fury and madness spewing out of him. "I can't take it! I can't take you! You're always crossing me! I'll do what I want! I want to see my mother. I'll just get out! I'm leaving!"

He raged up the stairs to the kitchen. I sat for a moment to get my breath and gain control. I closed my work on the computer. Then

I started quietly up the stairs as Tony was at the kitchen door to the garage, slamming around.

"I've already checked in at the Holiday Inn," he yelled, "I'm going."

"Sweetheart..." I started, and he slammed the door behind himself. Gone.

"Sweetheart..."

What could I have done? I drifted into a fragile sleep, the light still on beside the bed.

A thumping sound came from the front hall and I threw off the covers and ran to open the door. Tony was on his knees, head down, arms up, fists pounding the door so hard that when I opened it he literally rolled in and onto his back, arms and legs flailing uncontrollably.

"I'm going crazy! I don't know where I am! Where am I? I'm going totally crazy! Just kill me! There's no reason to live! You're driving me out of my mind!" His head whipped from side to side. His arms and legs stabbed at the air. Unearthly sounds came from his throat. I backed away, terrified. When he relaxed, I got down on my hands and knees and held him tight, whimpering, half crying, "You're home. It's your home. You're safe. I'm here. I'll never leave you. You're not going crazy. I love you. I love you."

Then fury struck again and I jumped back, afraid of his thrashing limbs. "Just kill me! I'm going crazy!" He grabbed at the railing, which divided the hall from the sunken living room. Then he let go, falling back and whispering, "Just kill me. I'm going crazy." We sat like that, crying and screaming for a long, long time. Eventually, Tony struggled to his feet and leaned on me. We shuffled to the bedroom. I took off his clothes and shoes and got him into bed. It was 3:30 in the morning.

"Why did I leave?" he asked, "What made me leave the house?"

"Just relax," I said, "It's over now. You can rest." I didn't want him to remember. But he did.

"You wouldn't let me see my mother!" Like a volcano, his rage came again, spewing out anger and confusion, his arms and legs jabbing like spears of lightning. I stood at a physically safe distance, but I felt burning heat flow over me.

"I'm exhausted," he said abruptly, and slept.

I did not. I threw on jeans and a sweatshirt and huddled at my desk with the phone. I needed help. I was afraid. My mother's words played in my mind, "You can handle it, Liz. I know you can handle it." Tony needed me now more than he ever had. I was his conduit to the world, to help, to comfort, to love. I was not helpless. I was not postponing my life. This was my life, the life I had chosen when I married him, and chosen again when I knew he was sick. I breathed deeply and shifted from a state of fear to a "handling-it" mode. Not waiting for offices to open, I picked up the phone in those early morning hours and left messages with doctors and organizations that could help.

By nine o'clock that morning, I had talked with our neurologist. When I described the incident to him he asked, "Had Tony been drinking?"

"No," I answered. No? He had been at the Holiday Inn bar for five hours. No? What was I thinking? Was I thinking? I had read and been told that Alzheimer's patients should stay away from alcohol, but I thought, what the hell? Life is over anyway, what difference could a glass or two of wine make? Now I knew that alcohol could have a devastating effect when combined with Alzheimer's.

By 9:30, our friend Don, a real estate person, was at the house to give me an appraisal on our property. I knew we couldn't stay here in a big house on an acre of lawn and garden, with no help or family nearby, and with Tony presenting such unpredictable behavior. Don and I stood in the driveway talking. I told him about Tony's illness and the frightening episode of the night before.

At 9:45, Tony came out into the sunshine, dressed, shaved, hair combed, smiling and greeting Don as though nothing had happened. I looked at him from across the driveway. I saw the man I knew so well, straight and tall and handsome. I was overcome with love and compassion for him. No one would guess he had a terrible, mind-destroying disease.

I felt confident enough to plan that trip to Holland where Tony was born and had lived until he was twenty-one. In Amsterdam, in between visits with his mother in the nursing home, we strolled along the canals, holding hands and stopping to eat Dutch pancakes and fried eggs with thin roast beef on fresh white bread. He showed off to me by speaking Dutch, German, and French. At night we held each other tight under a fluffy down comforter.

But it was evident that the dementia was progressing. "Don't tell me. I know. Our room is on the right," he said, as I steered him to our hotel room on the left. "Where are my, you know, my things?" he asked, looking for his underwear to pack in his already packed suitcase. "Oh, ha, ha! That's not where I want to go!" he said, opening the door to the hall, looking for the bathroom. He woke me in the night by sitting straight up in bed and remarking on the flowers climbing up the walls or the bicycle on the bedside table. He, who had traveled the world all of his life, was in a land more foreign than he had ever been, and I was the guide. "Well, you know, the women do everything nowadays," he excused himself as I ordered his meals, paid the bills and handled the tickets. Sadly, two weeks after our return, he forgot that we had seen his mother.

My level of acceptance of his illness grew, but I never knew how sick he was. He was always a little farther into the disease than my acceptance would allow. I was still looking for a plan of action, or some way to gain control of the chaos and to protect him from his disease. I accepted his behavior as it was at that moment and his life became my life. It was what I wanted to do, but it cost me.

For a few years, medication tempered Tony's rages of frustration, but inevitably his diseased brain deteriorated to the point where he had no control over behavior, no ability to recognize people or objects, and though he talked incessantly, no understanding of language. I found the help we both needed by placing him in an Alzheimer's nursing home. Two months later, when he was in the dining room of the facility, standing tall, greeting people and arranging chairs, a visiting Hospice nurse saw him and recognized signs of approaching death. Tony had developed an infection in a saliva gland which, if not treated, would spread and kill him.

He had shown me he wanted to leave years ago on that night he had slammed out the kitchen door. I knew he wanted to get away and be free of the disease, so this choice was not a difficult one. I allowed Hospice to help him go in peace and comfort.

Ultimately, of course, it was not my choice; his life was not in my control or his. Alzheimer's had taken over long ago. My choice was to provide love, respect, understanding and, lacking a road map, to seek out the best road, to soften the sharp curves and walk beside him as far as I could go.

Elizabeth Van Ingen was born in San Francisco and graduated from the University of California at Berkeley. She met her husband, a native of Holland, in Tehran in 1959, where she was teaching fifth grade at the American School. She now lives in the Denver area.

Homecoming

Deborah Miller Rothschild

The cloak of obligation and love that my husband had worn in his role as lifelong guardian to his retarded son slipped from his shoulders this summer, when Jude died. Now it lies crumpled around his feet, a tangle of emotions that needs examining before he steps free. But the weight of responsibility has lifted. The grief is easing. And we are facing a bittersweet holiday season that will be filled with love and relief, but also with tears.

Some days I think I can see all the way to Christmas. Finally there will be fall weekends when we won't feel guilty because we aren't visiting Jude. There will be no more Saturday mornings spent on the freeways, jockeying around eighteen wheelers while managing the butterflies in our stomachs and wondering what kind of mood Jude will be in when he greets us. We'll spend a relaxed Thanksgiving Day around our own dining room table with friends and family instead of eating with strangers in one of Lake Charles' low-end casino dining rooms, the only places open on holidays in that Louisiana town. On Christmas morning, for the first time, my husband and I will share a leisurely breakfast in our own house with carols playing in the background, instead of racing towards the rising sun to get to Jude before his mood blackens because he's become hungry waiting for us to arrive.

Jude, a Down syndrome man-child who could never grow up, unintentionally spent a lifetime controlling those who cared about him. When I became his mother almost eight years ago, Jude had the emotional maturity of a three-year-old. He expressed his wants and needs in three- or four-word sentences. He lavished expressions of affection or quick anger on anyone who happened to be nearby. And he adored his father.

At the time of Jude's birth forty-three years ago, Down syndrome children were routinely placed in institutions. So Jude waited for six weeks in a neonatal ward in Metairie, Louisiana before a place was found for him at Hammond State School. His fraternal twin was taken home to nurse at his mother's breast and be fully accepted as the younger brother by his older siblings. From the beginning, Jude's father understood his role as the protector and caregiver for his special child. Jude's mother responded differently. She chose to pull back and distanced herself from her retarded son. She saw Jude only once during the final twenty years of his life.

And so when I married Jude's father, I became Jude's mother. I would know him as a child only through stories of family visits to state schools, and through pictures of a grinning, towheaded youngster. By the time I met him, Jude lived in a school for retarded adults in Lake Charles, a blue-collar town that would become the center of my holiday celebrations and my once-a-month Saturday picnic destination.

Jude's behavior had become erratic. His moods and physical problems were controlled by a cocktail of sixteen different drugs, some taken several times a day. Often he would have an open wound in the middle of his forehead, the result of injuries he'd sustain while banging his head on the bathroom tile. He walked with a halting, Shrek-like gait and his eyes crossed. Unless he was reminded to close his mouth, his tongue often hung beyond his lips.

But despite his physical and mental limitations, Jude could work magic on anyone who spent time with him. When he was happy the sun shone and love beamed forth. Strangers stared, then smiled. Hugs were dispensed every few minutes. It was difficult to go anywhere in Lake Charles and not hear someone call, "Hey Jude."

However, thunderheads could pop up out of nowhere. Jude would become violent without warning. Although small, he was strong and could be dangerous. Because of his special needs and his mercurial ways, we could never bring him home. Our times with Jude were always spent in his world. Our relationship with him was based on love, but tainted by guilt and obligation, and filled with sacrifice. And now he's gone.

So this year the holidays will be different. For the first time Jude will be in our home, a place he could not visit during the time I knew him. His spirit will be freely embraced. And although there will be moments of sweet sorrow, we will be free to celebrate our extraordinary child whose gift to the world was unconditional love.

Deborah Miller Rothschild lives in Houston, Texas, and is a freelance writer, feminist, political activist and grandmother.

Mothering Mother
Carol O'Dell

Letter to Self

Dear Carol,

So far, you've been taking care of your mother for a year and a half. You've stuck it out through crazy times, angry times, tender times, through hospital visits and home health visits, and while everyone else comes and goes, you've stayed. You haven't had a vacation and no more than two days away this whole time.

I know you: I know that when your mother dies, you're going to feel guilty. You're going to think that you should have been kinder, not in a rush, that you should have done more with her, taken her more places, insisted the kids be nicer. I know you're going to miss her and wish that a million things had been different.

I want you to know you did the best you could. You remained faithful. You grappled with every decision. You let her into your life and your home, you and your family did what most people wouldn't even have considered doing, much less done. People aren't perfect, and if they try to be, then they're not real. We're not supposed to get it all right. Remember, you had to balance this with being a wife and mother. It's only natural to want to move forward and be more interested in your children—in those who are living. That's how the human race survives.

Remember, her emotions were always on an ever-widening pendulum, and Alzheimer's took them to frightening heights and devastating lows. You learned as a child that you couldn't trust her with your heart, although you kept trying. It just wasn't ever possible. That's okay. You know she loved you. And you loved her.

So go...love your children. Love your husband. Live life. Learn and grow and help others. Let it go.

Remember all the kindnesses—how Phillip built her apartment and put up her pictures, whatnots and books, how you tried to make it as much like home as you could, even before you did your own home. Remember stopping just to buy Klondike Bars for her. Remember the hot washcloths and how good she said they felt. Remember kissing her goodnight on her forehead, holding hands in the car and how much she loved getting her toes done. Remember how much she made you laugh and cry and want to scream.

You always knew you were alive with her. Remember.

Letter to Mother

Dear Mother,

I never wanted it to turn out this way. You, lost in confusion; me, overwhelmed and not knowing how to reach you. When you moved in with us, I was naïve enough to envision us sitting by the river, me holding your hand, you nestled under a lap blanket, and the two of us sharing memories of my childhood and your childhood. Somewhere in this idyllic dream, you'd doze. I'd feel the pressure of your hand loosen and I'd know you were gone. I would kiss your forehead and whisper, "I love you," as you began your journey home.

A fairy tale, I know.

The reality is that I tiptoe into your room each morning and hold my breath, watching for the rise of your chest. Not that I want you to die; rather I fear that you have. Your life seems futile. Your days consist of not much more than a series of meaningless actions and reactions. Are you now more driven by instinct? Do hunger and thirst and a need to be covered up and warm rule you in your wordless world? Am I trying to decide if your life is more or less valuable than mine? Who am I to say? Does this sound cruel? I don't mean for it to.

I wake each morning to view the remnants of your destructive night. I pick up the nightstand, the telephone that is no longer plugged in. There's a mound of clothes on the end of your bed that you've taken off the hangers. More work for me. You've taken everything off. Your skin is as white as the whole milk you drink, your eyes remain closed, shunning this world.

I thought you'd be different. I thought I'd be different. I didn't expect this. I miss you. I miss what little we had. I miss your humor, your laughter. You still laugh sometimes....

Integrity is what you do when no one's looking. I wonder how I measure up. It's not that I do cruel things—it's that I don't seem to be able to relax, to sit down with you, talk, read the Bible to you. I'm scared so I just keep on my feet. I want to help you make a scrapbook, watch some old TV show, anything that brings you a bit of pleasure. But it's too late. Those things no longer mean anything to you. Each day passes and my family needs me, but you need me too. I want to write, go for a walk, clean out the refrigerator, take a bath, anything to avoid you.

I haven't put you in diapers yet. You wet everything, and yet at least you still try to use the potty chair. I just can't do that to you—or me. I'm afraid the diapers will give you permission to give up. I know that day is coming, and I'm helpless to stop it, just another step in your descending world.

I guess what I resent the most is the endlessness of the situation. It's easy to be kind, loving and caring when there's a cut-off date. Cancer often makes people valiant. Families rally around loved ones and last wishes get fulfilled; but this just seems to run into oblivion. I fear the possibility of years of your existence, staring off into space, randomly screaming while I perform the duties of diaper changes, sheet and nightgown changes, wondering why.

I tell you I love you, especially at night. I try not to let a night go by without telling you. If you could hear me, understand me, step back to see this whole picture of our lives, I think you'd be proud of me, of us. We've made a good family. I love you still. I love that you loved me. I love that I had a mother.

Carol O'Dell's literary works have appeared in numerous magazines and anthologies including *Southern Revival Anthology*, *Margin Magazine*, *Atlanta Magazine*, *The Pisgah Review*, *Timber Creek Review* and *AIM—America's Intercultural Magazine*. She teaches creative writing and speaks on writing, caregiving and adoption issues. Her book, *Mothering Mother: A Humorous and Heartbreaking Memoir*, was released in April 2007.

Taking Care
Joann Price

Sometimes I wonder what happened to my life.

My constant concern is about my aging and very sick father. He didn't ask for this insidious cancer. He wonders, why me, why now? He wonders if the treatment is worth it, yet he isn't capable of stopping the process, because he is weak in mind and spirit. I see it in his eyes sometimes, the glazed look as someone speaks to him. He doesn't answer or he gazes down and finally says something that has little to do with the question.

How can I help him? Will my care matter? Will it make a difference? Am I doing enough? I know it's not about me; it's about him and my duty as a daughter. It is about my responsibility to the other members of my family. It is up to me to care for him so he lives longer and they can see him, talk to him.

I cannot take the place of my mother, who years ago died of lung cancer. Does he think about the care he tried to give her years ago? Does he remember what it is like to hop up every few minutes to provide something, even if it's just a smile or a slight touch on the forearm? Does he remember the worry when the discomfort is so plainly seen, or the pain becomes something that can't be managed any longer? Maybe he has wiped most of those memories from his mind. Who can blame him?

What will the next weeks and months hold? Will we, a year from now, look back, take a deep breath and remember, one more time, that we are glad it is over? Will it be one more time, thank God, that he is playing golf and going out to dinner? Or will I, weeks and months from now, be in the same place or in another place that I don't understand or wish for? Only God knows because it is obviously His plan.

I put my hands to my forehead and rub and rub. I rub my upper arms and shoulders, willing the aches to go away. I listen to him cough. I listen to his soft footsteps as he makes his way from the living room to the kitchen and carefully down the stairs. He isn't as sure-footed as he wants to be and I wait, holding my breath until he settles down again. When I wake in the morning I must bound from bed, in case he needs me and doesn't want to disturb my rest. I listen to the toilet flush, knowing he has made his way to the other side of his room, and glad that there is still a normal human act he can accomplish, and I breathe out again.

There is indignity to all this. There is some embarrassment to this caregiving, an embarrassment between a father and daughter. What will I have to do for him yet, to make it easier, swallowing the difficulty of it all for both of us, and plunging forward to do what must be done? I don't want to go there. But it isn't about me.

I'm not usually one to get teary-eyed. Lately though, that is exactly what I've been doing. I've been crying at night, as quietly as I can. I've cried in the shower. I've cried as I put laundry in the washer and dryer. It seems so overwhelming most of the time that it is easy to lose control as I watch him get weaker. I remind myself that selfishness is unbecoming. After all, when I was ill my parents took care of me. But should my life be turned upside down? Should everyone's life, but his and mine, go on, with only casual, occasional reminders of his plight? Why should my life be the one that is not the same? But those thoughts are just "poor me" thoughts, and I've no right to have them.

I'm afraid for him; I'm afraid he will suffer, and I will have to watch him, care for him, do what must be done, the most that can be done to help him not suffer. I know he is afraid. If I am to help him with that fear, am I allowed to have fears of my own?

Early this morning I went for a long walk. I looked up at the vast blue sky, taking deep breaths as I took my steps. I tried so hard to see the beauty, to bring the fresh air into my lungs, to ask God for His blessings, for patience, for forgiveness and mercy. Autumn leaves gently floated onto the street and onto the still green lawns. I relished the walk. I wanted to clear my head. I didn't want to return home. But I had to. And when I stepped through the back door into the kitchen, I mouthed the words, "Is he up yet?" My dear mate, who had already made the coffee and provided the multitude of prescribed medications, nodded yes, and by the look on his face, I knew that Dad didn't feel well. My mate's looks warned me to steel myself for another trying day.

Everyone knows that life is full of joys, sadness and frustrations. Life comes with love and hate. It comes with resentments, dangers, highs and lows. Both joy and sadness change the heart. I think about its shape. Is it round and smooth, or are the edges ragged, damaged? Do my tears change the shape of my heart and does my smile or my laughter heal it?

Some time, days or months from now, I hope to look back on this time and feel proud. I hope that I will think about these days with a strong faith, not one that is weak and dispirited. I hope that I will feel relief with strong deep breaths, rather than with shoulders that sag and shake with my moaning. Yes, relief, liberation, a hope for life's relief, certainly for him, and for me. I am left to wonder, and wonder some more!

Joann Price is a college English teacher, writer, reader, and a writing coach. Married for 30 years and a mother and grandmother, she hopes to move to the northwest coast where she can write and read by the sea.

Part VI
Humor

...laughter is the closest distance between two people.

— *Victor Borge*

A Crash Course: How to Be a Do-Right Cancer Husband

Marc Silver

I am a card-carrying member of the fraternity of clueless cancer husbands. When my wife was diagnosed with the disease in 2001, I didn't know what to say or what to do. Naturally, I relied on my instincts. Bad idea.

Let's take my reaction to Marsha's desperate phone call, sharing the news that the results of a callback mammogram had prompted the radiologist to tell her, "Sure looks like cancer to me." As she likes to remind me, I said, "Ew, that doesn't sound good." Not the kind of husbandly comfort she was expecting. (Although in my defense, it really didn't sound good.)

Now let's consider the way that phone call proceeded. We talked about what would happen next: a visit to the surgeon the following week to schedule a biopsy. We discussed whether to tell our two daughters about the tentative diagnosis and decided to wait until we had more definitive news. Then I said: "See you tonight honey." I hung up the phone. I stayed at work all day.

My wife thought she had called the wrong husband.

Okay, so I was not a Boy Scout. I was not prepared. I did not tell my wife, "I love you and we'll get through this together." I did not rush to her side. I did not leap into the fray. I played the denial game—maybe the radiologist is wrong. I stayed at the office because it was easier for me to deal with typical workplace stresses and strains than to plunge through the Looking Glass into the unfamiliar and unsettling place called Cancer World.

When I did rally to the cause, I overcompensated. I tried to fix things. I tried to cheer Marsha up, because I felt better if she was upbeat. But I didn't think about how she was really feeling.

Eventually, I learned from my mistakes. The number one lesson I learned: "Shut up and listen." That's the cancer husband's motto (although it works well for any husband in any circumstance, really). I do feel I need to clarify what I mean. Some misguided guys have misinterpreted the motto as "Shut up and listen to me"—proof that men really do think it's all about us. For the record, I mean: Shut up and listen...to your wife! Because she knows what she wants and needs. And you don't.

As it turns out, there are a lot of guys like me who need to master the art of shutting up and listening. I met dozens and dozens of them when I researched my book: *Breast Cancer Husband: How to Help Your Wife (and Yourself) Through Diagnosis, Treatment, and Beyond.* And I've met many more traveling around the country and speaking on the art of being a cancer caregiver.

For new members of the cancer husband club who'd like further advice, I'm happy to oblige. Here are 11 things you should not say to your wife or girlfriend after a diagnosis of cancer. These are all things that either I said or thought about saying, or that other real men really did say. Because you can't make this kind of stuff up. But you can learn from our mistakes.

1. You don't want those flowers—they're supermarket flowers.

A guy and his wife go shopping in the supermarket. She is a newly diagnosed cancer patient. She sees some flowers and admires their beauty and says she'd like a bouquet.

Her husband explains to her why she doesn't really want them. Because "they're supermarket flowers."

Here's the thing about flowers. They are a force for good in the midst of a terrible time. A colleague taught me this. She herself was a cancer survivor. She told me that when she was undergoing chemotherapy, her husband would have a big bouquet waiting for her at home after each session.

I followed his example. And to my amazement, the flowers made my wife feel better during the chemo months. I must confess, I really didn't understand why. I mean, they were just flowers.

Then I told this story to a friend, and she said, "Oh, you gave her flowers. How romantic!"

That's when I got it. Flowers aren't just flowers. They're a symbol of love. They conjure up memories of special occasions, of birthdays and anniversaries, of a time when you were courting your wife.

Dude, get her flowers.

And yes, even a bunch from the supermarket will do.

2. Cheer up, your odds of survival are 80 percent.

Quoting survival statistics is a common husbandly tactic. Gotta make her feel better, right? Most likely, wrong.

Coming to terms with a cancer diagnosis is a complicated process, fraught with emotions and uncertainty. Your wife may not be comforted by survival statistics. Because if eight of ten women in her situation survive, that means two of them won't.

It will be a boon for her if you let her share her fears and worries instead of dismissing them or trying to talk her out of them. In one study, a group of women who bitched and moaned about the awfulness of cancer coped better with the stress of treatment than a group of women who bottled up their negative feelings. These let-it-all-hang-out women even fared better than expected based on their initial prognosis. The psychiatrist who conducted the study says that it points up the damage that can be done by repressing emotions.

So, ladies: Complain away. And gentlemen: You don't need to tell her to snap out of it or otherwise try to fix things, as guys are wont to do. Sometimes all she wants you to say in return is, "Yeah, cancer really sucks."

3. You're doing great—you sure don't need any help from me.

Some women want to make it seem as if they can do it all: be a wife/mother/employee/cancer patient. They don't want to burden their husband; they act as if everything is under control. As a result, the husband acts as if everything is normal. He doesn't provide extra help at home, he doesn't go with his wife to doctor's visits and chemo sessions. Because look at her, she's handling it really well!

But if you're not by her side, she may come to feel that you really don't care about her. That's what one woman told me about her absentee husband.

Guys, even if she gives you a pass, or even if it seems her mother or sisters or friends are giving her all the help she needs, she needs your love and support, too. If you feel as if you're being shut out by all the other helpers, tell her that, and ask what you can do to meet her needs and ease her burdens.

4. Your real hair looked like a wig anyway. Or the runner-up: That wig looks better than your real hair.

My brothers, this is not what you say to your wife when chemotherapy robs her of her hair. Show a little empathy. Even if hair seems like a trivial casualty in the war against cancer, it is not. Many breast cancer survivors have told me that losing their hair was harder than losing a breast. A lost breast can be masked by a loose-fitting blouse. But a bald head is a potent reminder of everything that's gone wrong, and there it is, staring back at her in the mirror each morning.

The prospect of a bald wife may leave men speechless. Imagine yourself in this scene:

It's a Sunday morning. Your wife has had her first chemo. Her hair is thinning rapidly. You're fixing her pancakes for breakfast—hey, everything seems better with pancakes, even cancer. Your wife steps out of the room. It turns out she had a rendezvous with a Lady Gillette. She returns a few minutes later, as bald as Mr. Clean.

"Whaddaya think?" she asks.

What should you say?

The woman who told me this story said that her pancake-flipping spouse simply said: "You look beautiful to me."

His words are perfect. They're not wildly overstated. They're genuine. They're heartfelt. And I know exactly what he meant. With her smooth, egg-shaped head, my wife did look beautiful to me.

P.S.: If you're a fan of those hot baldies on *Star Trek*, now's a good time to let your wife know that a hairless pate can be a turn-on.

5. **Could you postpone your mastectomy until sailing season is over?**

Um, er, no! The husband who made this comment was tossed overboard by his new bride. You, sir, are not the boss of the cancer patient. She is the boss of you. Husbands need to understand that they are not calling the shots, picking the docs, or prescribing the treatment plan. Their job is to support the woman they love. She may ask what you think: Is this doctor the right one? Which chemo regimen do you prefer? But she will make the decision, not you.

6. A mastectomy isn't such a big deal.

That's how one woman's husband was making her feel as she contemplated the surgery. Angry at his lack of empathy, she asked him how he would feel if he were about to have a penis-ectomy. Gee, my wife asked me the same question! I tried not to take it personally.

The fact is, losing an organ—an organ tied to sexuality—is a big deal. Some women do have an easier time than others facing this surgery. One woman told me her breasts had served her well, had fed her infants, and now she was ready to let them go. But that's not how my wife felt when she faced the prospect of a double mastectomy. And it's not your job to tell her how she should be feeling.

7. I just gotta tell you how pissed I was when you *(fill in the incident)* last year.

A husband may be tempted to bring up every grievance from the past decade. A wife may share the same temptation.

A very wise radiation oncologist advises: Consider a moratorium on rehashing old wounds. Maybe you and your wife want to set ground rules: No revisiting any issues that are older than six months. And try not to say anything you'd regret if you're having a caregiver meltdown (which can happen, believe me).

When breast cancer strikes, you should be there for the woman you loved and married. I even heard of one couple that was proceeding with a divorce when the wife was diagnosed with cancer. The soon-to-be ex-husband stood by his wife, helping her deal with the difficult months of treatment.

8. I don't like starting something I can't finish.

That's what one guy told his wife when she said she was in the mood for kissing and caressing, but maybe not for sex. I mean, sheesh, she had just finished chemotherapy and radiation treatments. Can you blame her? And can you blame him?

Yes, you can.

As frustrating as it may be for the husband, there may be times during the cancer months when your wife wants to cuddle—and nothing more. By pulling away, the man is driving a wedge between himself and his wife. The loss of physical touch is one of the biggest losses you can suffer, one psychologist told me. Give her a back rub, massage her feet with some nice oils. These are important ways of keeping a physical connection at a time when life seems to be spinning out of control.

And yes, guys do like to finish what they start. Really, who doesn't? But you know what? Sometimes you can't. For the frustrated husband, I will pass on the advice that a truck-driving cancer husband shared with me: "Sometimes you have to be an owner operator."

9. Sex is going on vacation.

Cancer is definitely not an aphrodisiac (see above). But as my wife's oncologist gently told us: "You can maintain intimacy during this period." There may be times during the months of treatment when your wife is in the mood, and so are you. And for a few minutes you won't be thinking about cancer.

10. If it were me, I'd remember everything the doctor said.

If you go with your wife to doctor's appointments (and really, you should), you may be surprised that she doesn't remember half of what the doctor tells her. I remember thinking how I would surely be more tuned in if I were the patient. Then I came across a study showing that it's typical for patients with a critical illness to forget much of what the doctor says. And what the patient does remember often is not correct. Don't berate her; support her by taking notes at the visit or tape recording it, so there's a record that the two of you can review. It'll make your wife feel better. And it'll make you feel better, too. At a time when you're not sure how to be of help, here's a way to be tremendously useful.

11. That's behind us now.

This is how many men feel after their wife has finished her cancer treatments. It's back to normal! Honey, don't forget, today is car-pool today, and can you pick up my clothes at the dry cleaner while you're out?

Not so fast, buddy! As one woman told her husband, "I have to live with this every day for the rest of my life."

In the months after treatment ends, your wife may still not feel like herself. Sometimes, all the stress she's been through just catches up with her. She may be exhausted. Her body may remind her of surgeries she's had. If she went through chemotherapy, she may be suffering from what's called "chemo brain"—a diminished ability to multitask. It may be temporary, but it's very real.

In other words, cancer is not behind her.

Meanwhile, ahead of her may be a lifetime of worry. Not every day, but yes, she may well worry about recurrence.

Guys sometimes just don't get it. I heard a cancer survivor tell her surgeon that her husband expected her to pick up the lawn-mow-ing chores. Frankly, she didn't want to. The doctor offered to write her a prescription: No mowing for the next six months.

What's a husband to do? My friend, the answer lies in those four magic words I mentioned at the start of this essay. Maybe you should write them on your forehead in mirror-writing to serve as a constant reminder: Shut up and listen!

An editor at *National Geographic Magazine*, Marc Silver is the author of *Breast Cancer Husband: How to Help Your Wife (and Yourself) Through Diagnosis, Treatment, and Beyond*, named one of the top consumer health books of 2004 by *Library Journal*. In 2007, he was named a Yoplait Champion for his "extraordinary efforts in the fight against breast cancer." Marsha, a teacher, is today in good health. A lasting legacy of the cancer experience: when she tells him what to do, he shuts up and listens.

Whoosh!

Judy Kronenfeld

I am on my way to take Dad to the urologist. He has prostate cancer, which he has, of course, forgotten. It is a hot June morning in Southern California after days of marine fog. The jacaranda trees are scattering purple petals like wedding guests showering rice on brides and grooms.

When I get to the assisted living residence, he is not sitting in the chair where someone usually deposits him, this after I've called several times to remind them to remind him to be ready, which, of course, he forgets as soon as he is reminded. I check the other building, where he sometimes goes on his better days in search of some "action": Bingo, the occasional entertainer. Nope. A staff person emerges. Oops, he must have gotten on the bus taking residents to the drugstore. The executive director of the facility radios the bus driver. I drive back to the drugstore (where I have just been, to buy the denture tablets Dad forgets to use) and find him sitting in the facility van. The bus driver hands him over to me.

"We have a doctor's appointment," I say. "Whoosh," he says, his now most characteristic sound—a quick expulsion of breath through loose, slightly inverted lips, a kind of strong sigh. "I didn't know."

He is not entirely steady on his feet, as if he's forgotten for a second what walking is, or maybe he's forgotten where he is, this little shopping center a half-mile from where he lives now. He's wearing the same light-colored jeans—pee stained around the fly—that he was wearing a few days ago when my husband and I took him to dinner, and a few days before that, when I dropped by to give him a new darker blue pair I'd bought.

"Whoosh," he says, getting into the car awkwardly, feet all a-fumble.

"We're going to the doctor," I say.

"Oh. Any particular reason?" he asks.

I explain, roughly, about the prostate cancer.

"Oh, I didn't know," he says.

I turn off the radio that comes on as soon as the car starts. I tell him the upside: he'll just get a manual exam and a hormone shot to control the prostate problem. I don't discuss the radiation treatment possibly looming on the horizon, every day for eight weeks. When the radiation oncologist found out my father was 87, he told me no need for that, clearly doing a quick statistical computation. Chances of dying before the cancer kills him? Something or other percent. On the other hand the urologist, who actually looked into my dad's face during three appointments and who knows he's otherwise healthy, suggested that the optimal treatment is hormone therapy and radiation, though last time, he did say hormone therapy alone was a "good choice we have made together." I tried to decipher what that was code for.

Now, as we whiz down the boulevard under the blithe opulence of the jacarandas, I try to engage my father's long-term memory. I take his left hand in my right; his signature strong squeeze isn't quite forthcoming. What I want to know is how exactly he left Germany in 1934. I know his eldest brother Ben, now long dead, who stowed away on a ship and wound up in the U.S., was the one who arranged visas for my grandparents and my aunt and uncles, now mostly gone or ancient and sick. But it occurred to me that I don't know what the difficulties for a Jew, even a Jew with a visa, leaving the year after Hitler came to power, might have been. But I wind up feeding him more information than he gives me.

"I think I flew," he says.

"In 1934?"

"It must have been a ship, then," my father says. "Ben would know. Whoosh."

We stop for a long light; I have to take my hand back.

"And how is Duvid?" my father asks, maybe for the fifth time since I took him off the senior van, sweetening my husband's name, as he always does.

"David's OK," I say.

"And how are the children?" he says, also for the fourth or fifth time. I can feel his brain grinding through its gears. "How is Danny?" he asks. For a second I imagine my father imagining the children, now flung worldwide, in their beds, still at home.

"He's fine. He's still in Latvia doing research for his Ph.D. in Riga, at least some of the time."

"Oh, that's right," Dad says, "he's in Latvia." The words come off his lips with the aural equivalent of a vacant stare. The gears grind again, this time more protractedly. "And how is Mara?" he asks. "She's fine, right?"

"She's still in Morocco," I say.

"That's right. She's in Morocco." My daughter had called this morning. She's packing for her return to the U.S., anxious about the job hunt to come.

"But, they're both happy," he says. "I mean, they're happy."

"They're OK," I say.

"Whoosh," my father says. And then, as we enter the parking lot of the medical building, "Oh, we're going to the doctor."

"Yes."

"Any particular reason?" my father asks.

Dad opens the door and shows me into the urologist's office, like a well-mannered suitor on a date. There is no one in the waiting room. At first I am afraid they have scheduled him with the male nurse alone while the doctor is in surgery, which would be a problem since I really need the doctor to do that digital exam, to tell me that we can continue to make that "good choice" of hormone therapy "together," at least for now.

I am thinking, selfishly, of how much I want to get away for a couple of weeks this summer, and of how that will be impossible if David—even sweetened David—and I have to alternate taking Dad to radiation therapy every single weekday. Treatment which, despite assurances about how well it is tolerated (by the doctor, who hasn't experienced it), sounds nasty.

Partly in recompense for my thoughts, I reach across to give my Dad's thick, liver-spotted hand a squeeze. I stroke the left side of his bald head, his coarse fringe of white hair. I smile at him. He smiles back with a good-natured, self-effacing grin, as if we have just shared a mild joke at his expense. Reflexive immigrant ingratiation, even with his American-born daughter? Or the intrinsic sweetness of his nature? I still don't know. I give him one of the magazines I have brought along. He studies the cover carefully. Then he scrutinizes an ad on the flip side.

"And how are the children?" he asks.

I repeat what I've already said, adding a bowdlerized version of Mara's job anxieties. What the hell. "She's always had a good head on her shoulders," my father says. "She knows what to do. Right?" He still sees everything through the permanent rose-colored glasses of his immigrant generation.

Is this cheerful conversation really that different from all my conversations with my father, convinced that his American child and grandchildren possess all the ingredients for success and personal happiness? Now I'm not sure I remember if he's always been like this. How long will my own memories last before they go whoosh? Oh, but I do remember this: the optimism, his twenty-one-gun "smile and the world smiles with you" treatment, applied intensively, hands on, when either grandchild felt low. Odd thing is, it was pretty effective.

I wish my father could smile my son into calling him more often, even if their conversation dims more than it brightens, like a lamp with a bad connection.

Four years from now, on Valentine's Day, my son will have a "pure Grandpa moment": he will impulsively duck into a supermarket and buy boxes of chocolate for everyone he works with, the cooks, the drivers, his co-workers, and then go back and get a second box for the drivers, because there are so many of them.

Four years from now an East Coast cousin will call me up and tell me she must move closer to her grandchildren. She's just had dinner with my daughter Mara, and she'll say she covets the role Mara's grandfather had in her life. "He was the person with the 'single greatest influence,' your daughter said. I want that!"

But now it is June 2001, and we are waiting in the doctor's examining room, Dad in the one chair, me on an extra stool. "Well, when you write to the children, give them my very best," my father says, putting my magazine down with the pile on the waiting room table. I gently retrieve it.

I have told the male nurse who ushered us in that we hope we can still put off radiation if the doctor thinks the signs are good. He leaves and comes back with Dad's hormone shot, making a joke about schoolgirls sent out into the hall as he sends me out into it. "So, you want to go on radiation," the nurse says confusingly when he opens the door again to let me in. "No," I shake my head. "We want to put it off." "I didn't understand a word," Dad says, buckling his belt as the nurse exits. But he seems to sense my exasperation. He gives me that little self-effacing grin as he sits down again in the one chair. He has shaved erratically; there are long hairs under his chin, and some on his upper cheeks. "I feel as if I have one more baby," I say, to him, wiggling his nose with my fingers.

But I want to travel this summer, many summers, while I still can, I am thinking. I want to host gala June weddings for my happy children, when they marry talented, kind, and cute significant others. I want my father, his hair black, to hold the children's hands and mine in his vise-like grip, saying, "See, what did I tell you! They have good heads on their shoulders." I want him to be uncommonly gracious to my long-dead mother as they kvel over the grandchildren's mazel.

"I hope I don't act like a baby," my father says, turning up the smile wattage. I stroke his bald head. I remember, as a kid, how he let me pull his hair into a fluff on either side of his face; it was our Herr Doktor Einstein game.

At last the doctor arrives. He shakes my father's hand warmly; my father, who has just asked me again what office we are in and who we are seeing, nevertheless looks at him as if he were a long lost landsman; a fellow countryman, or the brilliant nephew recommended by a best friend. The doctor immediately launches into a well-meaning but tortured mode of medical speech that is, I think, a measure of his difficulty with being scientifically accurate in language that is understood by ordinary mortals. I glean that my father's blood work is good. I step out again while he does the digital exam.

When I come back, the doctor and I talk about fingers and how accurate they are, while my father, again buckling his belt, continues to beam beatifically. Reprieve, once again reprieve! From whatever it was that lurked in the future. I mumble about "quality of life...difficult decisions." The doctor goes on about the sound choice we have arrived at together, at least for the moment, and how we'll re-evaluate in four months, when we may well encounter a change in condition.

A phone rings in the examining room. "I'm not here," my father says gaily.

In the elevator on the way down, his arm in mine, I mumble about long-term decisions. "I'm not complaining," my father says. "I'm an old man. But I'm not complaining." We step out into the dazzling sun.

"I mean as long as you're helping me...."

"No point in talking now then," I say, pressing his arm a little tighter against me, as we negotiate the steps.

"Exactly," he says, righting himself from a slight falter as he transitions to flat ground. Together our eyes scour the parking lot; I spot the car that used to be his and we set off towards it.

"And how are the children?" my father says.

Whoosh.

Judy Kronenfeld's poems have appeared in *Poetry International, The Women's Review of Books, The Portland Review, Spoon River Poetry Review*, and in anthologies such as *Red, White & Blues: Poets on the Promise of America*. In addition to her poetry, she has published stories, essays, and a book of scholarship entitled *King Lear and the Naked Truth* (Duke University Press, 1998). She teaches in the Creative Writing Department at the University of California at Riverside.

(continued from page 194)

Advance Directives

Public opinion polls have revealed that close to 90% of adults in the United States would not want to be maintained on life-support systems without prospect of recovery. Yet a survey of emergency department patients found that 77% did not have *advance directives*, the legal documents, such as the living will, durable power of attorney, and the healthcare proxy, which allow people to convey their decisions about end-of-life care ahead of time. Some surveys show that most people think it is the physician's responsibility to initiate the discussion about advance directives. Yet, in surveys of physicians, they felt that patients should start the discussion. In the end, it would be ideal if both the physicians and the public made an effort to start the conversation.

Advance directives provide a way for patients to communicate their wishes to family, friends, and healthcare professionals and to avoid confusion later on should they lose the capacity to express those wishes. A good example of an advance directive tool is *The Five Wishes*. Five Wishes lets your family and doctors know:

1. Which person you want to make health care decisions for you when you can't make them.

2. The kind of medical treatment you want or don't want.

3. How comfortable you want to be.

4. How you want people to treat you.

5. What you want your loved ones to know.

Primary care physicians are in an excellent position to speak with patients about their care preferences because of the therapeutic relationship that already exists between them and their patients. Hospice and palliative care specialists are trained and experienced in conducting these discussions. In general, it is preferable that the patient brings a close family member, caregiver, or friend along for these discussions so that the patient's care preferences can be witnessed and any potential surprises or conflicts can be explored with the family.

Such discussions have particular urgency in patients who are showing early signs of cognitive impairment, because advancing dementia may rob the patient of the ability to communicate their wishes. In older persons with existing cognitive impairment or dementia, it is important to assess both their current degree of decision-making capacity and any evidence, written or verbal, of previously stated preferences.

The Big Picture

In discussing advance directives and care preferences, each person should explore his or her own values—what is important, what makes life worth living, and what makes life intolerable. The clinician should help the patient identify and set realistic goals, then direct treatment decisions according to these goals. It is important to evaluate whether the patient would prefer to focus on length of life or quality of life if faced with a serious or terminal illness. In older persons who have chronic conditions that are not immediately life threatening, there is more time to explore these issues and to modify decisions over time. Outlining the available treatment options (for example, the probability and extent of response to treatment, duration and quality of extended life, anticipated side effects), identifying patients' short- and long-term goals and needs, uncovering their expectations about therapy, evaluating their coping strategies, and identifying their support networks are critical components of this discussion.

The Details

Having thought about and discussed the big picture or overall goals, it is then important to consider specific life-sustaining treatments such as *cardiopulmonary resuscitation* (CPR), artificial nutrition and hydration, and *mechanical ventilation* (artificial breathing machine). It is reasonable for patients to ask physicians to review the potential indications for such therapies and to offer, if possible, an appraisal of the outcome in their situation.

For physicians and health care professionals, it is critical to consider the person's cultural, ethnic, and religious background while eliciting patient preferences for care. For example, it is fairly well known that Jehovah's Witnesses will not accept blood transfusions, even in the face of life-threatening bleeding situations, but may want all other invasive treatments. Such differences can make a patient unwilling to accept a physician's recommendations and can make a physician angry at the patient's resistance to those recommendations. With patience and training, however, it is usually possible to uncover these beliefs and negotiate treatment plans that are acceptable to all concerned.

Caregiving

Informal caregivers are family members or friends who provide care to chronically or seriously ill persons. Most are women, elderly, and have health impairments and needs themselves. If they were to be paid for their work, the cost would amount to billions of dollars per year. It doesn't matter how many hours each week are spent providing support.

Caring for a family member or friend is not easy, nor is it something most of us are prepared to do. Learning about being a caregiver may help you provide the care your friend or loved one needs.

There are many aspects to caregiving that one might not think about. These include preparing oneself for giving care, planning ahead and making a checklist, providing actual care as well as coordinating care. In addition, a caregiver will need to know about helpful services within the community, knowing when to get help, and obtaining information about finances and advance care planning. Very often, caregivers are so busy or stressed that they forget to take care of themselves. Recent data show that caregivers who perceive caregiving to be stressful are at higher risk for medical and psychiatric illnesses themselves. Caregivers cope (or not cope) in different ways, as illustrated in the following quotes:

"I feel privileged to be able to take care of my father. He made me who I am, and I owe it to him."

"My mother has been dying of dementia for 10 years! I never thought it would be like this. I'm having a breakdown. When she dies, she's taking me with her."

"Even though we were divorced, when my ex was diagnosed with cancer, I had a spiritual awakening that I should care for him. Those were some of the best times we had, more honest sharing than ever."

There are professional caregivers as well, such as paid home health aides or clinical nurses' aides. These aides may form strong bonds and relationships with the patients and their families over time, and can become emotionally or physically affected by the work they do. This is a disenfranchised group because their grief is often unrecognized or unaccepted, since, after all, they are getting paid. Increasing attention is being paid to this at-risk group.

Because hospice and palliative care recognize the patient and the caregiver as a single unit of care, these specialties provide more support and services to care for the caregiver, while the caregiver takes care of the person who is ill.

Summary

Palliative care is a team approach to providing the best quality of life for people with serious illnesses and their families, regardless of prognosis. It does so by addressing the whole person rather than organ systems, relieving physical and emotional suffering, and promoting open discussions of goals of care. Hospice shares the same philosophy and provides comprehensive, team-based services for the last stage of life, and follows the bereaved caregiver for continued support.

Our healthcare system is in a crisis because it is geared towards providing acute care, while we are now transitioning to a world where people live with, and die of, chronic illnesses. Their care requires ongoing evaluations of goals of care, and changes in plans of care. Yet the healthcare system fails to reward or reimburse for good communication, teamwork, or continuity of care.

Palliative care and hospice have been growing as a field and will continue to grow, as baby boomers age in place and medical technologies create more situations for fragmented care. The Centers for Medicare & Medicaid Services (CMS) will need to re-evaluate the hospice benefit for the 22nd century, and probably extend the time period to say, 12 months, to allow for greater use of this comprehensive program. CMS will need to take the lead to restructure and build in reimbursement for those elements of healthcare that are in jeopardy, such as clinical communication, coordination of care, teamwork, and continuity of care.

Dr. Cynthia X. Pan, MD, AGSF, FACP, is the Medical Director for Queens County for Hospice Care Network (HCN), a certified not-for-profit hospice organization serving families and patients in Nassau, Suffolk and Queens counties in the State of New York. HCN is one of the oldest, largest, and most respected hospice organizations in the State of New York. As Medical Director, Dr. Pan provides home visits to patients who are homebound, administrative leadership and medical oversight to an interdisciplinary staff, and educational leadership to doctors and nurses in training.

She received a Bachelor of Arts degree in biology from Harvard/Radcliffe and a medical degree from Stony Brook University. She completed her Primary Care Internal Medicine residency at the University of Rochester in New York and Geriatrics Fellowship training at Harvard Medical School's Division on Aging. She was a faculty member of the Departments of Geriatrics and Medicine at the Mount Sinai School of Medicine in New York City from 1997 to 2006. She served as Director of Education at the Hertzberg Palliative Care Institute at Mount Sinai from 1999 to 2006. Dr. Pan is board certified in internal medicine, geriatrics, and hospice and palliative care.

Dr. Pan was the recipient of an HRSA Geriatric Academic Career Award focusing on educational leadership in geriatric palliative care. She is also a member and currently Chair of the Ethnogeriatrics Committee at the American Geriatrics Society (AGS).

Her professional interests include the education of students and housestaff in effective and compassionate care of patients with complex and serious illnesses across different cultural groups and disciplines. She is an active clinician and teaches medical students, housestaff, and various discipline members about geriatric, palliative care and hospice.

Life With Dax

Derek Neeld

My ten-year-old son Dax was diagnosed with autism at the age of four, and life with him has been an adventure. Dax was two when he started making "The Line" each night before bed. Dax had an enormous collection of Matchbox cars and trucks. He loved this collection and played with it all over the house and yard. Before bedtime, he would take this collection and make a very straight and ordered line of certain cars and trucks placed end to end. Everything in The Line had a specific place. Though Dax had dozens of cars and trucks in his collection, he always knew if one was out of place or, worse, missing. And since he played with them constantly, both inside and outside the house, it was a rare night when at least one or two weren't missing.

A missing car or truck meant a furious tantrum until it was found and properly placed in The Line. Dax was completely nonverbal at this time, so if a car or truck were missing, he couldn't tell us which one it was. To make matters worse, there were cars and trucks in the collection that didn't make it into The Line on occasion and the composition of The Line varied from week to week. We'd go through the process of searching high and low for the missing car or truck, bringing those we found to Dax for inspection, hoping we had found the right one. Most often we hadn't and the search continued. This could take hours. If The Line wasn't complete, no one would get any sleep.

The Line lasted about a year. I wish I could say why Dax quit making it or that my wife Crystal or I did something that caused him to give it up, but I can't. Dax either outgrew The Line or simply got tired of it. We weren't sad to see it go.

Dax was three when he decided to be a dog. We had three dogs kept in the backyard and these were Dax's best friends. One morning after breakfast, Dax went outside to play with them. When Crystal looked outside to check on him a few minutes later, he was gone. She called me and together we searched the backyard but found nothing except his discarded clothes. We weren't concerned at first: not answering our calls wasn't unusual and taking off his clothes was nothing new, either. However, we began to worry after searching for him without success.

We were close to panic when Dax finally showed himself. Completely naked, he came crawling out from underneath the house. In his mouth he held an old squeak toy we had bought for the dogs. Crystal and I were both too shocked to do anything other than laugh. We tried to grab him, but he took off back under the house and sat near the opening, just out of arm's reach. We tried pretending to walk off, and when Dax poked his head through the opening, we'd rush over and try to grab him. We were always too slow. Finally, Crystal had an idea. She went into the house and returned a few seconds later with a box of doggie treats. Waving a treat in front of the opening, she was able to coax Dax out just enough for me to grab him. He growled and barked but I was able to drag him out.

That was the first time Dax decided he was a dog, but not the last. For the next year he sometimes urinated outside like a dog, leg hiked and all, and licked people on the face when he was happy. Once, he even tried to mount me while we were playing horsie. That was an awkward moment, let me tell you.

Dax was in first grade when the first really big challenge came. We had fought tooth and nail to have Dax put in an inclusive classroom and things had gone smoothly for the first few months. Everyone was telling us how well Dax was doing and how hard he was trying. Then something happened that threatened all that: Dax started hating white pants. Anytime another student or teacher wore white pants Dax would become violent towards that person. He would lunge and charge, push them out of their desk or tear at their clothes.

He never seriously hurt anyone, but it was becoming a significant problem. It got to the point where Crystal and I were called to the school almost daily because Dax had gone after someone wearing white pants. The principal told us that if we couldn't get this problem under control, Dax would have to be removed from the classroom on a permanent basis.

We tried story boards. We tried time out. We tried corporal punishment. We tried everything. We even tried to convince Dax that there was no such thing as white pants, that the offending pants were cream colored instead of white. He didn't buy it.

Things were approaching the critical stage. Other parents had started to complain to the school about Dax's outbursts. Finally, Crystal took the gloves off. She decided the next day that she wasn't going to like whatever color pants Dax wore. She was going to go with him to school and act ugly to him all day because of the color of his pants. She was good at it too; I almost felt sorry for Dax. And you know what? It worked. Dax gained understanding by being put in the position of the people he was hurting. Crystal made Dax tell her what she could do to not be upset by the color of his pants. By having to think of ways to help Crystal, he learned to deal with his own problems. Dax's behavior improved. He had some relapses, and when he did Crystal would repeat her act the following day. Slowly but surely, the incidents slowed until Dax finally quit attacking people who wore white pants.

We've haven't had to worry about white pants in a long time. Sometimes it takes creative steps to produce the desired result. Persistence and thinking outside the box always prevail.

Between the ages of four and eight, Dax had an adventurous streak and a disturbing lack of fear (which I understand is common in autistic children). Even when he was closely supervised, it wasn't unusual to find him lying in the middle of the street, standing on the roof or jumping out of a tree. Crystal and I had to turn our house and backyard into a domestic version of Fort Knox. Ladders were kept strictly under lock and key. Buzzer alarms were placed on the front door so we would know when it was opened. We built an eight-foot-tall cinder block fence around the backyard and installed the gates that couldn't be opened from inside. We even had to put an alarm on Dax's bedroom door because he liked to sneak out of his room in the early morning hours and get into mischief. Our house was like a prison. It was the only way to keep Dax out of trouble.

Dax was five when he began to intentionally injure himself during tantrums. He would run face-first into a wall or jump head-first off the couch. Other times he would punch himself in the face. It was horrifying just how dedicated Dax could be to hurting himself. Tantrums, at their worst, could stretch into hours. To keep Dax safe during these episodes we practiced pressure restraint, lying gently on top of him or hugging him tightly until the fit passed.

Unfortunately, this type of behavior wasn't just limited to our home. He had these tantrums at school as well. They were especially bad when they first began, since his teachers and aides were woefully unprepared to deal with his fury or his determination to self-injure. Thankfully, Dax eventually grew out of this behavior. By the time he was seven, self-injury was rare and it was gone completely by the time he was eight.

There were times Crystal and I would resent Dax for his behavior, especially if he caused a scene in a public place and embarrassed us. Dealing with the emotional backlash of these feelings was particularly rough. We'd cry over feeling that way about our son, no matter how fleeting the emotion was. But life with Dax can also be funny. The social skills of autistic children can lead to humorous and/or embarrassing moments, and Dax's skills have provided quite a few. One day we were in the grocery checkout line. A rather heavyset lady was in front of us. She accidentally backed into Dax and when she turned to apologize, Dax responded with, "You're fat." Just as blunt and loud as can be. The look she gave me could have peeled paint off walls.

Another time we were having a family dinner at Red Lobster. Dax was standing in his chair so he could better see the large aquarium across the room. The waiter had just come to take our order when Dax got an itch near his private parts, one he couldn't quite reach through his pants. Still standing in the chair, he pulled down his pants and underwear and began to scratch himself. I don't know which caused the bigger scene: Dax doing a striptease or Crystal diving across the table to pull his pants back up.

We live in an oil and mining town, so people often have the "blue collar" appearance while in convenience store lines or in the bank on payday. Lately, whenever we are next to someone who appears dirty, Dax will make a great show of sniffing the air, followed by gagging sounds and asking: "What stinks?" Subtlety is obviously not a skill he possesses.

One day at school, Dax told a girl he had a crush on, "We're going to get married and mate like killer whales." Too much Discovery Channel, I guess.

One aspect of autism we found extremely difficult to deal with was the treatment we got from others. Friends and even family members distanced themselves from Dax. They were always afraid of setting off a tantrum and were scared to be around him. It really hurt when we'd leave him with his grandparents, only to have them bring him back home ten minutes later. Looks and comments from strangers hurt as well. People would glare at us when Dax was having a fit, as if to say we were horrible parents who had no control over our child. We frequently heard comments like, "If that were my son…." We'd want to scream, "You don't understand!" Sometimes we'd feel alone, especially when friends were talking about their children performing in school plays and such. It was often easy to imagine we were the only parents in the world with a child like Dax.

But we got through it all. No matter how bad it was, we got through it.

We've had many more experiences and adventures than the handful we've shared here. It's been an exciting ten years. It has been a very rewarding ten years and, at times, a very difficult ten years. But we wouldn't trade them for the world.

Derek Neeld lives in Carlsbad, New Mexico, where he and his wife Crystal raise Dax, their ten-year-old son diagnosed with autism. They treasure each day with Dax, good or bad.

Dad's Private Police
Catherine A. Johnson

Just over a year ago, my father began telling strange tales of being kidnapped and secretly videotaped. He talked much like my mother did in the later stages of her struggle with Alzheimer's disease. I was sure we were heading down the same path. The staff at his care facility noted the behavior and lived with it; they could do nothing for him. It was only when he was admitted to the hospital with chest pain that I was able to help bring my Dad some peace and comfort.

He suffered a mild heart attack and was taken by the staff to the hospital. I received the call at 7:30 A.M. that morning and headed to the emergency room. Removing an 87-year-old man from his familiar surroundings, routines and medications is a dicey matter, to say the least. The hours it took for admission did not help matters. While we waited, my father told me that a man, sitting outside the window of the examination room, was cleansing his blood through a tube in his arm. The man he was referring to was working at a computer screen. My father was amazed and thrilled with this new blood cleaning technology.

When he was finally taken upstairs to coronary care, I went outside to call my siblings. Upon my return, everything had changed. He was no longer passive and cooperative. The unfamiliar room had become a dangerous place to him. I found him sitting on the edge of the bed, pale and wide-eyed, taking swings at the nurses to keep them back.

"Oh, Cath!" he cried. "That man over there [pointing at his roommate], he has drugs and booze and he has people in the hall coming to kill me!" When I tried to calm him, he persisted. "Cath, you don't know…you have to call the police, get security!" How it hurt to see him so very terrified. He calmed down only when I promised to stay with him and keep watch.

All afternoon I sat and watched him as he lay sedated and huddled under his blanket. My hero, the strongest man in my life, was a terrified little boy who whispered while pointing at people who weren't there. It broke my heart. My presence was not enough to calm him and neither were sedatives.

The stories he told persisted, each one more wild and frantic than the previous. Upon my return from getting something to eat, he was pointing out the door at a man in the hall who was sneaking up to kill him. He said there were people outside the third floor window with machine guns; he urged me to duck. I wanted to ease his fears but it was apparent that even my staying with him all night was not going to do it. The nurses decided to move him to a single room near their station, in the hope of giving him some relief. That is when I saw a possible band-aid for his notions of being the target of gangsters.

My town is home to a very large prison and this hospital cares for its inmates. In the next room was an inmate being watched by two prison guards, both in uniform, packing weapons and badges. Could I? Would they? What the heck. I called to the two rather large young men and the smaller one came to the door.

"Listen, my 87-year-old father is being moved to this room because he is sure someone is out to kill him," I explained. "If I told him you were here to protect him as his personal bodyguards, would you go along?"

The officer grinned. "Sure, be glad to."

So when they wheeled my father's bed down the hall, I had them stop the bed just outside the door and said, "Dad, you asked me to call the police, now I want you to see." I waved the officers over. They stood on each side of his bed, one bigger than the other, hands on guns, badges shining. "Dad, these officers are here to protect you. They are your own personal police and will be here all night."

"Yes, sir, that's right," said one as he tapped Dad's knee.

My Dad's eyes welled with tears as he looked over at me. "Good boys.... Good boys," he said in a cracking voice. I thanked the officers as my father was wheeled into his new room. I doubted whether this helped Dad sleep—I am sure he was still watching the windows—but he did know he had someone to call who had guns at the ready to protect him. And for me, well, the important thing was that I'd done something, and when you watch a loved one suffering, you just want to do...something.

While she and her husband of 32 years were raising three teenage children, Catherine A. Johnson also helped care for her mother, who died from Alzheimer's in 2000. Since her mother's death, writing has helped her to express her emotions and preserve precious family memories. She lives in Michigan.

Afterword

Caregivers Seeking Advice: A Doctor's Prescription
Rosemary Laird, MD, MHSA

Life demands only the strength you possess. One feat is possible—
not to have run away.

—*Dag Hammarskjold*

What do caregivers value most in the doctors who care for their
loved ones? Early in my career, I thought I knew the answer: that
the doctor can cure their loved one. But over the years, as my
training and clinical practice became more focused on geriatrics
and Alzheimer's disease, I have learned otherwise. Caregivers tell
me that what they need reaches beyond cure. Caregivers need a
doctor who listens to their loved one's values and wishes, and
bases his or her medical opinions on that critical foundation. This
helps caregivers achieve a level of comfort and confidence that
they have done all they can. But how do you find doctors who listen? How do you find other caregivers who can help raise your
comfort and confidence? Over the years I have learned a great
deal from the caregivers of my patients. Two of them help us here

as we look at the steps you can take towards comfort and confidence in your caregiving.

Barbara is a leading educator in our community. One day, she called and asked for help. Her mother's health had taken a frightening and unexpected turn for the worse. Then 71 years old, her mother had been living and thriving independently in a nearby town. She became ill that winter with what was diagnosed as the flu. Barbara had not visited, due to her mother's concern that the illness was "contagious." They kept in touch by phone until Barbara began to suspect that her mother was not recovering as quickly as she should. Disregarding her mother's protests, Barbara went to her mother and found her in poor physical condition, not taking her prescribed medications and not eating properly. Barbara's mother was admitted to the local hospital's intensive care unit, where Barbara heard the dreaded estimation that "we can't do anything but wait and see." Barbara's mother spent weeks in the hospital, but happily was eventually discharged and able to move in with another family member to complete her recovery. Today she is back home and living independently once again, but now with weekly—and sometime more frequent—visits from her dutiful daughter.

Months later, Barbara and I reflected on those uncertain days. I was surprised when she told me of her greatest fear during the ordeal: "What worried me was being the one responsible for making sure Mother got the all the possible care. But the healthcare professionals involved in her care were focused exclusively on the lifesaving part of the work, which left me on my own. If she was going to die, even after everything possible had been done for her, then it was out of my hands. I wanted to make sure I learned what I needed to know. But instead of relying on the medical professionals caring for mother, I had to rely on my friends and colleagues for advice on what to do."

As I listened to Barbara talk about her mother's ordeal, I was struck by the source of Barbara's fear: that she wasn't doing all she could for her mother. She worried that she wasn't asking the right questions, finding the right doctors, keeping her mother away from medical errors, and making the right decisons. Professional caregivers often believe that the the caregiver is looking for "the cure," when just as often the caregiver understands that there is only so much that medicine can do. More important to the caregiver is the assurance that all has been done to give their loved one the best care and, if possible, additional days, months, or years of *what their loved one would consider a quality life.* But as caregivers and patients become immersed in the complicated and chaotic world of a hospital or health system, such clarity is elusive at best.

I recall thinking, if only I were one of the doctors involved in caring for Barbara's mother, not just a collegial advisor. It was not because I felt the outcome for Barbara's mother would have been any better, but because Barbara had no one listening to her concerns and needs. The healthcare system's endemic lack of support for caregivers was increasing Barbara's already significant stress. But over the years caregivers have taught me it is possible to mitigate the uncertainties that lead to emotional turmoil. You can take steps to prepare for a loved one's health crisis and manage care through it, by creating a therapeutic alliance with the doctors and the other healthcare professionals who make up what seems like an impenetrable healthcare network.

Step 1: Get Close to Your Loved One

To caregivers, nothing is more comforting than knowing they are carrying out their loved one's wishes when making life-altering decisions. If you don't currently have this type of relationship, don't wait for a crisis to hit! Well before a health crisis occurs, make sure you fully understand two things. First, know your loved one's wishes in the event that decisions need to be made on his or her behalf. Second, know what insurance and financial resources are available. Include all important family members in these discussions, and determine well ahead of time who will be responsible for making decisions. If a crisis does come, you will be well prepared to help with the complicated decisions that are likely to be faced.

Given the complexity and fast pace of the healthcare system, it is best for anyone admitted to a hospital due to an acute health crisis such as a stroke, hip fracture, or serious illness to have someone with them from the time of admission and, afterwards, for as many hours a day as possible. If you or another close family member cannot personally get there, enlist the help of a neighbor, friend from church, or other relative who can get there quickly. If these options are not available to you, you may want to consider hiring a professional geriatric care manager. These professionals are typically nurses or social workers and can be hired on a fee-for-service basis to provide a wide range of support and care services. They can be invaluable as your loved one's advocate, a knowledgeable resource about healthcare resources, and your "eyes and ears" in the local setting. Care managers can also help local caregivers continue to work while managing the health needs of a loved one.

Jan, a registered nurse, holds a master's degree in business administration and worked her way up the ranks to be vice president of a well-respected health maintenance organization in our community. Her father was diagnosed with Alzheimer's disease and ultimately needed to be placed in a nursing home. When her mother was diagnosed with Alzheimer's disease a year after her father's death, Jan found herself a caregiver again.

Her mother was fortunate to have had a long-term primary care physician who provided a vital focus for care. "My parents were among his first patients. He was very supportive. He would pull me into the office and tell me what the next steps would be. His mom had Alzheimer's disease and he explained things to prepare for." But no matter the preparation, there are always unexpected turns of events that can change plans in an instant. Jan found it invaluable to have a trusted geriatric care manager who could help direct and manage her mother's care while Jan attended to the day-to-day duties of her work and immediate family. Find geriatric care managers in your local area by checking with your local Area Agency on Aging or www.eldercare.gov.

Step 2: Connect with the Caregivers

The more connected and visible you make yourself to those caring for your loved one, the better off you both will be. Healthcare is like anything else in life: a personal relationship and good rapport can make everything go a bit more smoothly. Do your part to communicate well, respect the time of others, and keep focused on the needs of your loved one. Keep staff aware of how to best contact you. A word of caution: don't get caught in the HIPAA (Health Insurance Portability and Accountability Act) roadblock. HIPAA is a federal law which may prevent your loved one's healthcare providers from disclosing to you information about your loved one's condition. Make sure you are listed as someone who can receive information about your loved one. Most often, a medical release signed by your loved one will be needed to enable healthcare providers to deliver information about your loved one's health status to you. If there is no formal authority, such as a living will or durable power of attorney for healthcare, some healthcare settings will accept a verbal release from your loved one.

Step 3: Educate Yourself: Learn the Facts and Ask for the Options

Too often, the overwhelming newness and complexity of the healthcare system causes us to become passive. It is sometimes easier to simply accept the advice and opinions given to us by the professionals. But in some instances, those on whom we rely offer only routine suggestions. Be proactive and ask them if there are any alternatives available. As examples: Can rehabilitation be provided in my mother's home instead of in a rehabilitation hospital? What would we need to do to have her go home? What do the different facilities available for this kind of care offer? Is there a superior facility across town for this type of problem? Often, referral patterns are set by geography and patient preference for being close to home. If you are open to going "where the care for this type of problem is best," let that be known. It might be the place down the street, but it might be an hour away. Being open to finding the most skilled and successful providers of the type of care you need will serve you well, though it can necessitate some additional work on your part.

Step 4: Plan Ahead

Always look down the road and plan for the next steps. Tomorrow will come more quickly than you think, and you do not want to be forced into decisions due to time constraints. This can be challenging when the next steps are not entirely clear. But even if all the details of the type of care that is needed are not yet known fully, you can often get a lot done ahead of time. For example, if you know your loved one will need additional help once they are discharged, review the financial resources available and discuss preferences on location and type of facility. Clear up differences of opinion within the family before you have to make final decisions. You can then narrow down options as the clinical status and the "next-step" needs of your loved one become clearer.

Step 5: Stay Calm and Focused...No Matter What They Throw at You

A typical caregiver lament I have heard over the years has been, "I never knew one day to the next what was coming... I wanted to walk away." Of course, these moments pass and reality comes back into focus. The best course of action is to keep yourself focused on the key outcomes for your loved one. Is the goal to get to rehabilitation? Is the goal to get back home? Is the goal to have your loved one free of pain? Keep these goals in mind and remind the professional care team of them, directly and often, if you see they are moving in a direction that does not support these overall goals. Be careful not to let emotions sidetrack your efforts.

For any caregiver, the stress level is enormous. You must be prepared and steel yourself to stay calm, get facts, and deal with whatever arises. At times, there is no room for emotion; often, emotion must wait until after the decisions are made. To make decisions you need to have good information. The professionals don't always recognize the caregiver's need for information, so caregivers must ask for it. "They seem to be in their own world of doing what they do," Barbara told me. "I had to decide on how to be proactive and not be seen as bothersome. Sometimes I had to ask two or three times for information, but I was not leaving there without it." Never raise your voice, never be mean, but be persistent.

Following these steps can help you feel that you've done your best to navigate the healthcare system and find the answers needed for making good decisions with, or on behalf of, your loved one.

Finding That Special Someone

"Navigating the healthcare system" is the phrase most often used to describe how one gets the healthcare and supportive services needed. The healthcare available in the United States is among the most sophisticated and specialized of any in the world. Unfortunately, the financial structure of insurance-based healthcare has led to decentralization and marked complexity in how one actually gets care. Thus, while there are superior services available from which to choose, we bear a heavy burden of identifying, locating, coordinating, and paying for the services we need.

I get more and more calls like this: "I know you aren't my mother's doctor, but I don't know where to turn, who to ask...." When someone I am not caring for professionally asks me to help them navigate the healthcare system for their loved one, I often start by asking them who they count on that will take the time to listen and understand their questions and concerns and then render valuable medical opinions. Unfortunately the answer is all too often, "No one." If you find yourself in that situation, I urge you to resist the understandable urge to run away! Return to Step 1. Listen and learn your loved one's needs and desires. Persistently seek the same from the professionals you encounter. Don't stop until you find someone who will both listen and advise, in that order.

Dr. Rosemary Laird is the founding Medical Director of the Health First Aging Institute (www.eldercare.health-first.org) located in Melbourne, Florida. Established in 2002, the Aging Institute sponsors clinics for geriatric consultation, memory loss, and primary care, and educational and support programs for caregivers. Affiliated programs include Leeza's Place, a community resource center for patients with early memory loss and their caregivers.

Dr. Laird received her medical degree from Georgetown University School of Medicine and completed residency training in Internal Medicine at the University of Chicago. She received a master's degree in health services administration from and completed a Geriatric Fellowship at the University of Kansas.

Afterword

When Angels Appeared:
Narratives in Complementary
Medicine

Ooi-Thye Chong, RN, MPH, L.Ac.

Remembering

It was the late 1970's; I was fresh out of nursing school in London. My eldest sister, Chiw Siam, the sole caregiver for our mother, telephoned from Malaysia to inform me that things were not looking good: our mother was dying of cervical cancer, was in pain and crying out in the middle of the night. I booked the next available flight home.

In the course of my training, I had come across patients who were dying, but I was still unprepared for the emotional and psychological challenges of facing the death of my mother. I arrived home to find her bed in the sitting room—in our culture, a sure sign that things had taken a turn for the worse. My heart skipped a beat and my throat tightened to suppress a cry when I saw how my mother had become shrunken and diminished—a shadow of herself.

I sat by her, feeling utterly devastated and helpless. In a weak voice, she asked me to take her to the hospital; she believed and hoped that there she would be cured. She was not ready to die. She had worked hard all her life and, now that her children had grown into useful contributing members of society, she wanted to enjoy the fruits of her labor. But we did not want her to die in the hospital. I told her I was home to take care of her. I can still see her face now—the disappointment, sadness and perhaps fear. The image still haunts me.

Chiw Siam and I nursed our mother until she died. When we washed and changed her, I saw tears of pain on her face. Many years later, I realized that these were tears of emotional pain and sadness as well as pain from her cancer and immobility. But she did not once complain and endured it as gracefully as she could. At the time I had neither the professional maturity nor the emotional depth to understand the complexities of her pain. Now I know that she would have been deeply comforted and soothed by being held or by gentle rubs to the limbs, feet, scalp and back. These simple measures—touch, love and tenderness—would have benefited her enormously. Over the course of my career I have learned that sometimes just being present with an ill person or just holding her hands in silence can be more meaningful and comforting than any words.

In life and in death, my mother profoundly influenced my work, but it took me years to understand it. Taking care of my mother was a terribly painful yet enriching experience. There were times when I experienced great comfort and succor as well as a profound sense of guilt and regret. The comfort and succor came from knowing that I had done my best and from being with her during her last days. The guilt came from a nagging doubt that I had not done quite enough for her, that I had failed her in so many ways. My husband reminds me that my mother had Chiw Siam and me to nurse her, and that itself must have been a great comfort to her. I hope that she had a good death—for there is such a thing as a good death.

The Gift of Forgiveness

For years after my mother's death, I would dream about her: her pain; her body disintegrating in front of me; conversations in which she reproached me. But one particular dream was the most important. In it, I was killed in a volcanic eruption and buried deep in the soil. I was crying and begging someone to ask my mother to dig me out and take me home. In my waking hours I tried to make sense of this dream—it seemed to me that this dream was telling me to break free of my guilt. Interestingly, once I accepted this interpretation, I started to have a whole new set of recurring dreams. In these dreams, I had wings. I flew gracefully and lightly with incredible joy and freedom. I felt the breeze brushing gently against my skin. I could breathe easily and feel the air filling my lungs. The sensation was exhilarating. When I awoke from these dreams, I always felt comforted, happy and light as a feather. I knew then that my mother had "taken me home," that I no longer needed to feel guilty and I could accept my mother's death as part of a natural cycle of life and death. Through these dreams, I learned over time to embrace life fully, not to judge myself too harshly, to be compassionate and to forgive myself for all the things that I feel I did not give my mother. This personal experience was to reverberate throughout my life and especially in my work with patients diagnosed with cancer.

Opening One's Mind and Heart

The next great lesson of my professional life occurred 15 years after my mother's death. I had the great good fortune to work with the late Dr. William R. Fair when I accepted a position as the Director of Haelth at the Complementary and Alternative Medicine (CAM) Center in New York City, founded by Dr. Fair.

Dr. Fair had been a buttoned-up, conservative and traditional physician who was not open to the notion that CAM therapies had anything to offer patients. But in 1995 he was diagnosed with colon cancer. After exhausting what the best of conventional medicine had to offer, he wanted to know what else he could do for himself. Out of desperation, he turned to CAM. It marked the beginning of a major change in his attitude and life. When he started to open his heart and mind to the possibilities, miracles happened. Dr. Fair began a journey of discovery and healing.

He started a routine of yoga, meditation, exercises, acupuncture and herbs. Gradually, he began to feel better physically and emotionally. Following this routine not only enhanced the quality of his life but also changed his view of health and illness to one in which emotions play an integral part in healing. By then, he fully understood that CAM therapies could be of great help when conventional medicine failed. Importantly, he believed these two worlds need not clash, and that one need not wait until one has exhausted conventional medical treatment before using CAM therapies. Rather, they could work hand in hand, bringing the best of both worlds to the patient.

I gained much knowledge and, I daresay, wisdom working with Dr. Fair and the patients at Haelth. I carry within myself the lesson of keeping my mind and heart open to possibilities. I was convinced by my experience that integrating CAM into conventional medicine could be done and was of great benefit to the patients. Dr. Fair was a perfect example of "integrative oncology," using the best of conventional and CAM therapies to achieve the best possible result. When Dr. Fair passed on in 2002, it was six years after conventional medicine had predicted his end.

Listening and Receiving:
The Power of Connection

One of my many roles as the Director of Program Development at Haelth and as Manager of the Integrative Oncology Program at St. Vincent's Comprehensive Cancer Center in New York is to provide health consults to our patients. The aim of such a consult is to design a program of CAM therapies that answers the question, "What else can I do for myself?" It is also an excellent opportunity to establish a therapeutic relationship with the patients, a relationship that, studies have shown, is critical to the success of the healing process.

Many of the patients I work with have some form of cancer and are at various stages of treatment. They are often scared, anxious and under tremendous stress. Some are desperate to live a few more months so their babies or toddlers can grow old enough to remember them. Their struggles remind me so much of my mother's situation when she was critically ill. They share with me their pain, their hopes and how their cancers have affected them. I listen. I offer sympathy and suggestions. I dare to share their pain; I have seen the comfort it brings to patients when someone is present and listening. There is something very healing and enriching, for both parties, when connections are made and a therapeutic relationship established, a skill I did not possess when I was taking care of my mother.

In her book *Kitchen Table Wisdom*, Rachel Naomi Remen talks about the power of listening and learning to receive what is being said. By so doing, we connect with our patients and ourselves, and begin to establish a therapeutic relationship. Listening with care, concern and kindness has to be one of the most powerful notions that I've come across. Below are some examples of patients with whom I have had the honor of working who have benefited from this simple idea.

Tom telephoned me when he was diagnosed with a brain tumor. He was experiencing difficulties in finding an oncologist with whom he felt comfortable. He was very distressed and frightened by the diagnosis. He wrote the following about his telephone encounter with me:

> ...she knew that the diagnosis had disturbed me emotionally and she listened carefully and quietly while I talked...what an immense help Ooi-Thye was to me. She was the first person to show me that kindness could exist in this frightening world of illness.... She was the

first person to say things to me that helped me through my ordeal and set me on the road to healing. She gave me the gift of comfort and wise counsel when facing catastrophic illness.

Howard was a physician who was diagnosed with late stage prostate cancer. He and his wife Liz had heard how well Dr. Fair was doing and wanted to follow in his steps. They planned to spend the weekend in the city so that Howard could implement the program of CAM therapies that was to be designed for him after his consult with me. He would follow the program when they returned home.

Ten minutes into the consult, I realized that Howard was avoiding eye contact with me and had not uttered a word. Liz did all the talking and she even answered questions that I had addressed to Howard. Realizing that he did not want to participate, I changed the direction of the conversation. I gently inquired if he was all right and if he would like us to terminate the consult. I clarified that if we were to continue, I needed him to actively participate in the process. He was surprised but he agreed. He proceeded to tell me how much he enjoyed food and good wine; how he loved to cook; how convivial and enjoyable it was to sit down with good company to a delicious meal and a nice bottle of wine. When he was describing the kind of foods and wines he enjoyed, his face lit up; it was like a ray of sunlight had just penetrated the room. Then Liz mentioned that she had hired two macrobiotic chefs to cook for him. I saw an abrupt change in Howard's demeanor. He was adamant that he was not going to eat a macrobiotic diet no matter the health benefits! There then ensued a somewhat heated exchange between husband and wife. I had to call a truce. I pointed out that food is a gift to our senses: visual, auditory, taste and smell, and provides nourishment to our body and soul. To eat with resentment, I said, is counterproductive. One could still eat healthily and enjoy the experience without going macrobiotic. Eventually, they agreed to consult with our dietician to explore how this might be achieved. They looked relieved because this had been a subject of conflict in their household.

Based on our consult, I recommended Reiki and restorative yoga to address anxiety and enhance a sense of well-being, as well as acupuncture for fatigue and pain. On his first day at Haelth, Howard received a massage and a session of restorative yoga as well as a consult with the dietitian. He left looking relaxed, even happy. With humility and a big smile he bowed when he bade us goodbye.

Both he and Liz felt that they were being heard. He was assured that he need not follow a macrobiotic diet. She was reassured that he could eat healthfully and still enjoy his food.

Gathering the Flocks Home and the Body/Mind Connection

According to Chinese medicine, the *Shen*, or the spirit, the very essence of the self, nests in and is nurtured by the heart space. When the Shen is in its residence, there is tranquility and harmony. During traumatic times such as having a cancer diagnosis or in the face of possible death, the heart space is shattered and cannot provide a peaceful residence for the Shen. Thus like a bird, it flees its nest. When this happens, the person experiences profound disharmony, depression, emptiness, fear, restlessness and anxiety. I often witnessed this phenomenon in our patients.

Alicia was a 23-year-old woman, diagnosed with ovarian cancer. She exhibited all the symptoms mentioned above as well as constant nausea from aggressive chemotherapy. The anti-nausea medications had not worked very well for her and she was retching constantly. She looked very uncomfortable, nervous and exhausted. I asked if she would like to do some work with me. I gave her an abbreviated explanation of the above discussion on the Shen and some images to work with: because of the intensities of what she was experiencing, her Shen could not rest peacefully at home, i.e., in her heart, causing a tremendous amount of turmoil. It was as if a fox has been let loose in the chicken coop, creating chaos and consternation. The short but powerful exercise we were about to do would help to gather the flocks home to rest. In short, she would be calmer in body and mind and less nauseous. I asked her to get herself in a comfortable position and gave her the following instructions:

1. Put the right hand over the heart/diaphragm area.[1] This calms the heart and mind and sends an invitation for the "flocks to return home."

2. Put the left hand over the *Tantian* (the area below the umbilicus and the pubic bone).

3. Breathe normally but more slowly, and as she breathed out, to imagine she was breathing out her anxieties, fears and frustrations. As she connected her energies and balanced them, she would feel calmer, more centered and less nauseous.

4. At the same time, I put my hands on both her feet, with fingers over her ankles and soles.[2]

We practiced this for about 20 minutes: gradually her breathing slowed down and her body relaxed. Miraculously, her nausea disappeared. When I left the room, she was fast asleep.

I returned 30 minutes later to check up on her. She was still asleep. When she awoke, I suggested to Alicia that she practice what we had just done together. The skill was hers to use whenever and wherever she felt anxious, scared or in turmoil. It is a simple, powerful and calming technique.

The Best of Both Worlds

In my experience, traditional medicine often holds the answers to problems when conventional medicine has none. This is why having an integrative therapy program within a conventional medicine setting makes so much sense.

A Case of Liver Qi Stagnation

Susan, 60, was undergoing chemotherapy for colon cancer. She was extremely anxious, at times depressed and had difficulty sleeping. She complained of pain in the right hypochondrium. She had intermittent difficulty inhaling and a feeling that her airway was obstructed. All medical examinations and relevant tests were inconclusive. She was referred to me, since conventional medicine could not find anything that could explain her symptoms.

After taking her pain history and doing *hara* (abdomen) palpation, it was clear that she had what Chinese medicine would call *liver qi stagnation* and *plum pit qi*. Liver qi stagnation is a very important and common pattern that typically presents as a feeling of distension, or tightness, over the liver area, along with moodiness, a feeling of being "wound up" and at times depression. The pulse is often wiry.[3] Plum pit qi is related to liver qi stagnation, and it is caused by emotional problems giving rise to a feeling of constriction in the throat. This feeling appears and disappears according to the emotional state being experienced.

I explained to her and her oncologist that what she was experiencing was, in Chinese medicine, a well-recognized and common pattern of disharmony and could be treated successfully with acupuncture. Both she and the oncologist were initially skeptical, although they did not say so at the time. Her symptoms decreased after the first acupuncture treatment and the problems were resolved after the third. She also reported feeling generally better and her breathing was much improved. She became a "convert" and thereafter received acupuncture on a regular basis.

Angels Appeared When...

Samantha was in her 20's when she died from lung cancer. She was in a tremendous amount of pain which did not respond to medication. I arrived to find Samantha in a fetal position and hardly able to speak or interact, only to request acupuncture. Her oncologist supported the use of acupuncture.

The results were dramatic. Samantha sat up a few minutes after the needles were removed. She was pain-free. She continued to receive acupuncture twice a week as well as some pain medications when necessary. For the rest of her short life, the combination proved very effective.

I remember very clearly her desperation, anger and frustration. I also remember how different she was during the short period of time when she was pain-free. I could see a glimpse of the spunky, smart and funny young woman that she was before the cancer got the better of her. I was deeply affected by her death.

A Pair of Tuning Forks?

Reiki therapy is the laying on of hands to restore balance to the body and mind. One can liken the hands to a pair of tuning forks that re-establishes a sense of balance and harmony. It is a great supportive healing therapy because it is gentle and non-invasive. It has no medical contra-indications. It is, therefore, an invitation to wellness.

My clinical experience informs me that Reiki is effective in reducing pain and anxiety. Ninety-seven percent of the patients who report pain and/or anxiety experienced improvement in their symptoms after receiving Reiki treatment. Below are patients' comments on the treatment:

"It was relaxing and helped the pain."

"I feel better balanced, more centered after Reiki. During the session [there was] noticeable dissolving of tension and pain."

"I feel more relaxed/more tolerant of the treatment."

"Nausea gone."

"A state of calm was induced; I could feel myself giving myself over—a very salutary experience."

"Definitely feel more balanced!"

It is easy to understand why Reiki is so popular with our patients. It is comforting and it is effective in reducing pain and anxiety.

Lessons Learned: Personally and Professionally

People often ask, "How could you work with people who are so ill," or "How do you do it without being burned out?" Or they will say, "I could not do what you do." The truth is that when it comes down to it, one can and one will. This is because working with those in need is not just about giving. It is also about receiving, connecting and healing. As I alluded to earlier, when you give, you almost always receive, sometimes in ways you never anticipate. It is an immensely satisfying profession and a great honor for me.

In the face of huge challenges and suffering, many of my patients show great dignity and strength. They teach me lessons that no book or degrees could ever give me. They teach me about myself as well as about life and death: life is for living and death is part of the natural order of things in the universe. I have learned what it takes to live one's life to the fullest, to move on and not get stuck with life's minutiae.

Yes, of course, I am deeply affected by the patients with whom I have worked. After all, I am human and do grow fond of them. When they have good news, I rejoice with them. When the news is bad or when a patient dies, the sense of loss is devastating. But I do not see this as inappropriate. Rather, it shows that I am capable of feeling the emotions of loss and sadness. It shows the humane and human side of me. Life is precious, fragile and yet strong at the same time.

At the end of each day, when I leave work for home, I always check in with myself: have I made a difference in at least one patient's experience of her illness? If I have, I have been successful in what I set out to do every day: to bring the best of CAM therapies into conventional medicine in order to make a positive difference in the patient's experience.

Ooi-Thye Chong, RN, MPH, L.Ac. is a registered health visitor (U.K.) and registered nurse (U.K., U.S.). She earned a master's degree in public health from Columbia University and a bachelor's degree with honors in social psychology from Sussex University (U.K.). She is also a national board certified and New York State–licensed acupuncturist. Her background is rooted in health promotion and integrative medicine. In London, she was a key team member of a primary healthcare practice with the first integrative program in the U.K., opened in 1980 by the late Princess Diana. She has also served as a researcher for the World Health Organization and a nurse educator for the United Nations.

She has served as the Director of Program Development of Haelth, a complementary medicine center founded by Dr. William R. Fair. She created and currently oversees an innovative integrative medicine program at St. Vincent's Comprehensive Cancer Center in New York City. Her focus is on enhancing the patients' sense of well-being and making a significant difference in their experience of their illness. She has a private practice in personal health consultancy and acupuncture.

While the patients described in this essay are real, their names have been changed to protect their privacy.

1. In Chinese medicine this area and the Tantian are important energy centers.

2. In my experience, and without fail, this practice of just holding the patients ankles and soles is very calming, soothing and grounding. There is an acupuncture point at the upper third of the sole which is translated as "Heart of the Soul."

3. In Chinese medicine there are at least 27 types of pulses and they are one of its most important diagnostic tools.

Resources

On the following pages you will find information on some of the foremost organizations focused on support for the caregiver, including information on the organizations written about by contributors to this book. These and many more may be found by visiting www.thehealingproject.org.

Caregiver Resources

American College of Physicians
190 N. Independence Mall West
Philadelphia, PA 19106-1572
Telephone Number: (800) 523-1546, x2600 or (215) 351-2600
Website: http://www.acponline.org/patients_families/end_of_
life_issues/cancer/

Provides a home care guide for patients with advanced cancer.

Family Caregiver Alliance
180 Montgomery Street, Suite 1100
San Francisco, CA 94104
Telephone Number: (415) 434-388 or (800) 445-8106
Fax Number: (415) 434-3508
Website: http://www.caregiver.org/

Family Caregiver Alliance provides information, education, services, research, advocacy and support to sustain the work of families nationwide caring for loved ones with chronic, disabling health conditions.

Health First Aging Institute
6450 US Highway 1
Rockledge, FL 32955
Telephone Number: (321) 434-4300
Email: info@health-first.org
Website: www.eldercare.health-first.org

The Aging Institute sponsors clinics for geriatric consultation, memory loss, and primary care, and educational and support programs for caregivers.

Leeza's Place/Leeza Gibbons Memory Foundation
3050 Biscayne Boulevard, Suite 605
Miami, FL 33137
Telephone Number: (888) OK-Leeza
Website: www.leezasplace.org
Email: info@leezasplace.org

Centers where caregivers of individuals with memory disorders can find resources, information, guidance and a sense of community.

National Alliance for Caregiving
4720 Montgomery Lane, 5th Floor
Bethesda, MD 20814
Email: info@caregiving.org
Website: http://www.caregiving.org/

National Alliance for Caregiving provides support to family caregivers and the professionals who help them and raises public awareness of issues facing family caregivers.

National Caregivers Library
901 Moorefield Park Drive, Suite 100
Richmond, VA 23236
Telephone Number: (804) 327-1112

Website: http://www.caregiverslibrary.org/

An extensive online library for caregivers.

Well Spouse Association

63 West Main Street, Suite H
Freehold, NJ 07728
Telephone Number: (732) 577-8899 or (800) 838-0879
Fax Number: (732) 577-8644
Email: info@wellspouse.org
Website: www.wellspouse.org

The only national organization focusing exclusively on the needs of spouses caring for a chronically ill and/or disabled husband, wife or partner.

Alzheimer's Foundation of America

322 Eighth Avenue, 7th Floor
New York, NY 10001
Telephone Number: (866) AFA-8484

Provides optimal care and services to individuals confronting dementia, and to their caregivers and families, through member organizations dedicated to improving quality of life.

Financial Help with Prescription Drugs

American Cancer Society

Prescription Drug Assistance Programs
Telephone Number: (800) ACS-2345
Website: http://www.cancer.org/docroot/home/index.asp

Association of Community Cancer Centers

11600 Nebel Street, Suite 201
Rockville, MD 20852-2557
Telephone: (301) 984-9496
Website: http://accc-cancer.org/

Provides contact information for reimbursement assistance programs for oncology-related services.

The Leukemia & Lymphoma Society
Southern Regional Office:

11 Canal Center Plaza, Suite 111
Alexandria, VA 22314
Telephone Number: (703) 535-6650
Fax Number: (703) 535-8163

Midwestern Regional Office:

9435 Waterstone Boulevard, Suite 190
Cincinnati, OH 45249
Telephone Number: (513) 583-8900
Fax Number: (513) 583-8143

Western Regional Office:

1550 E. Missouri, Suite 204
Phoenix, AZ 85014
Telephone Number: (602) 532-0404
Fax Number: (602) 532-0407

Provides a prescription drug co-pay assistance program for patients with myeloma, Hodgkin's lymphoma, non-Hodgkin's lymphoma and acute myelogenous leukemia.

Multiple Myeloma Research Foundation
383 Main Avenue, 5th Floor
Norwalk, CT 06851
Telephone Number: (203) 229-0464
Email: info@themmrf.org
Website: http://www.multiplemyeloma.org/

Operates pharmaceutical reimbursement assistance programs for multiple myeloma patients.

Information on the Medicare Prescription Drug Benefit Program

American Cancer Society
Website:http://www.cancer.org

Health Insurance Information

National Coalition for Cancer Survivorship
1010 Wayne Avenue, Suite 770
Silver Spring, MD 20910
Telephone Number: (301) 650-9127 or (888) 650-9127
Fax Number: (301) 565-9670
Email: info@canceradvocacy.org
Website: http://www.canceradvocacy.org/resources/

Legal Assistance

American Cancer Society
Website: http://www.cancer.org

Provides help dealing with financial and legal matters related to your cancer experience.

National Coalition for Cancer Survivorship
Website: http://www.canceradvocacy.org/resources/guide/

Provides information on employment rights for cancer survivors.

Financial Assistance

CancerCare
275 Seventh Avenue, 22nd Floor
New York, NY 10001
Telephone Number: (800) 813-HOPE (4673)
Fax Number: (212) 712-8495
Email: info@cancercare.org
Website: http://www.cancercare.org/

Cancer*Care* provides free, professional support services to anyone affected by cancer, including people with cancer, caregivers, children, loved ones, and the bereaved.

National Cancer Institute
NCI Public Inquiries Office
6116 Executive Boulevard
Room 3036A
Bethesda, MD 20892-8322
Telephone Number: (800) CANCER
Website: http://www.cancer.gov/cancertopics/factsheet/Support/financial-resources

Provides listings of financial resources information for people with cancer.

National Coalition for Cancer Survivorship
1010 Wayne Avenue, Suite 770
Silver Spring, MD 20910
Telephone Number: (301) 650-9127 or (888) 650-9127
Fax Number: (301) 565-9670
Email: info@canceradvocacy.org
Website: http://www.canceradvocacy.org/resources/

Provides listings of financial resources information for people with cancer.

Assistance with Lodging

American Cancer Society Hope Lodge
Telephone Number: (800) ACS-2345
http://www.cancer.org/docroot/SHR/content/SHR_2.1_x_Hope_Lodge.asp

A network of 22 Hope Lodges offering free, temporary housing facilities for cancer patients who are undergoing treatment.

Travel Assistance

Corporate Angel Network
Westchester County Airport
One Loop Road
White Plains, NY 10604-1215
Telephone Number: (914) 328-1313
Toll-Free Patient Line: (866) 328-1313
Fax Number: (914) 328-3938
Email: info@corpangelnetwork.org
Website: http://www.corpangelnetwork.org/

Corporate Angel Network's mission is to ease the emotional stress, physical discomfort and financial burden of travel for cancer patients by arranging free flights to treatment centers, using the empty seats on corporate aircraft flying on routine business.

Government Health Organizations and Resources

Administration on Aging (AoA)
Administration on Aging
Washington, DC 20201
Telephone Number: (202) 619-0724
Fax Number: (202) 357-3555
Email: aoainfo@aoa.hhs.gov
Website: http://www.aoa.gov/about/contact/contact.asp
Office of the Assistant Secretary for Aging: (202) 401-4634
Public Inquiries: (202) 619-0724
Eldercare Locator (to find services for an older person in his or her locality): (800) 677-1116

Part of the United States Department of Health and Human Services, AoA is one of the nation's largest providers of home and community-based care for older persons and their caregivers. Services include home-delivered meals programs or nutrition services in congregate settings, transportation, adult day care, legal assistance or health promotion programs.

U.S. Department of Health and Human Services
200 Independence Avenue, S.W.
Washington, D.C. 20201
Telephone Number: (202) 619-0257 or (877) 696-6775
Website: http://www.hhs.gov/

HHS is the United States' principal agency for protecting the health of all Americans and providing essential human services, especially for those who are least able to help themselves. Their website includes a directory of resources and information on protecting the privacy of personal health information.

DisabilityInfo.gov
Website: http://www.disabilityinfo.gov

DisabilityInfo.gov is a comprehensive online resource designed to provide people with disabilities with quick and easy access to the information they need on numerous subjects, including benefits, civil rights, community life, education, employment, housing, health, technology and transportation.

Food and Drug Administration (FDA)
5600 Fishers Lane
Rockville, MD 20857-0001
Telephone Number: (888) INFO-FDA (463-6332)
Website: http://www.fda.gov

The FDA is the United States government organization that regulates the nation's drug industry. It maintains information on all drugs and treatments that are available to consumers in the United States.

healthfinder.gov
P.O. Box 1133
Washington, DC 20013-1133
Telephone Number: (800) 336-4797

Email: healthfinder@nhic.org.
Website: htpp://www.healthfinder.gov

Healthfinder.gov is a key resource for finding the best government and nonprofit health and human services information on the Internet.

National Institutes of Health (NIH)

9000 Rockville Pike
Bethesda, MD 20894
Telephone Number: (301) 496-4000
Email: NIHinfo@od.nih.gov
Website: http://www.nih.gov

NIH is the primary federal agency for conducting and supporting medical research.

Office of Special Education and Rehabilitative Services

U.S. Department of Education
400 Maryland Avenue, S.W.
Washington, DC 20202-7100
Telephone Number: (202) 245-7468
Website: http://www.ed.gov/about/offices/list/osers/

Committed to improving results and outcomes for people with disabilities of all ages.

Online Resources

Hospice and Palliative Care Association of New York State

http://www.hpcanys.org/about_hp.asp

The Hospice and Palliative Care Association of New York State (HPCANYS) is a not-for-profit organization representing hospice and palliative care programs, allied organizations and individuals that are interested in the development and growth of quality, comprehensive end-of-life services. The Association provides a strong, active voice for patients and their families. It advocates for public policy—both state and federal, and legislative and regulatory—that promotes accessible, quality end-of-life care.

Legacy Writer

http://www.legacywriter.com/livingwill.asp?src=g12healthcare
directivese

Helps people complete advance directives, such as living wills.

The Five Wishes

http://www.agingwithdignity.org/5wishes.html

Helps you express how you want to be treated if you are seriously ill and unable to speak for yourself. It is unique among all other living will and health agent forms because it looks to all of a person's needs: medical, personal, emotional and spiritual. Five Wishes also encourages discussing your wishes with your family and physician.

National Hospice and Palliative Care Organization

http://www.nhpco.org/templates/1/homepage.cfm
HelpLine: (800) 568-8898.

NHPCO's Vision: A world where individuals and families facing serious illness, death, and grief will experience the best that humankind can offer.

NHPCO's Mission: To lead and mobilize social change for improved care at the end of life.

Caring Connections

http://www.caringinfo.org/

An initiative of NHPCO that provides a wide range of free materials about end-of-life care. A good site for consumer education about hospice and palliative care.

Center to Advance Palliative Care (CAPC)
http://www.capc.org/

CAPC provides healthcare professionals with the tools, training and technical assistance necessary to start and sustain successful palliative care programs in hospitals and other healthcare settings. CAPC is a national organization dedicated to increasing the availability of quality palliative care services for people facing serious illness.

Growth House, Inc.
http://www.growthhouse.org/

Provides a portal as the international gateway to resources for life-threatening illness and end-of-life care. Its primary mission is to improve the quality of compassionate care for people who are dying through public education and global professional collaboration. Its search engine gives you access to the Internet's most comprehensive collection of reviewed resources for end-of-life care.

American Academy of Hospice and Palliative Medicine (AAHPM)
http://www.aahpm.org/index.html

The Academy is the professional organization for physicians specializing in hospice and palliative medicine. Membership is also open to nurses and other healthcare providers who are committed to improving the quality of life of patients and families facing life-threatening or serious conditions. Originally organized as the Academy of Hospice Physicians in 1988, the Academy began with 250 charter members and has grown to well over 3,300 in 2008.

The National Family Caregivers Association (NFCA)
http://www.thefamilycaregiver.org/about_nfca/

The NFCA educates, supports, empowers and speaks up for the more than 50 million Americans who care for loved ones with a chronic illness or disability or the frailties of old age. NFCA reaches across the boundaries of diagnoses, relationships and life stages to help transform family caregivers' lives by removing barriers to health and well-being.

familydoctor.org
American Academy of Family Physicians
11400 Tomahawk Creek Parkway
Leawood, KS 66211-2672
Telephone Number: (800) 274-2237 or (913) 906-6000
Fax Number: (913) 906-6075
Website: http://familydoctor.org

This website is operated by the American Academy of Family Physicians.

The Merck Manual of Medical Information
Merck & Co., Inc.
One Merck Drive
P.O. Box 100
Whitehouse Station, NJ 08889-0100
Telephone Number: (908) 423-1000
Website: http://www.merck.com/mmhe/index.html

The world's most widely used textbook of medicine. This edition is developed specifically for patients and caregivers. Information is available online for free.

Medical Professional Associations

American Academy of Pediatrics
141 Northwest Point Boulevard
Elk Grove Village, IL, 60007
Telephone Number: (847) 434-4000
Website: http://www.aap.org/

An organization of 60,000 pediatricians committed to the attainment of optimal physical, mental, and social health and well-being for all infants, children, adolescents and young adults.

American Geriatrics Society
The Empire State Building
350 Fifth Avenue, Suite 801
New York, NY 10118
Telephone Number: (212) 308-1414
Email: info@americangeriatrics.org
Website: http://www.americangeriatrics.org/

A not-for-profit organization of 7,000 health professionals devoted to improving the health, independence and quality of life of all older people.

Gerontological Society of America
1220 L Street NW, Suite 901
Washington, DC 20005
Telephone Number: (202) 842-1275
Fax Number: (202) 842-2088
Email: geron@geron.org
Website: http://www.geron.org/

A nonprofit professional organization with more than 5,000 members in the field of aging, the Society provides researchers, educators, practitioners, and policy makers with opportunities to understand, advance, integrate and use basic and applied research on aging to improve the quality of life as one ages.

Finding Physicians, Hospitals, and Clinics

**Health Resources and Services Administration—
Bureau of Primary Health Care**
Website: http://www.bphc.hrsa.gov/

This organization will help you find a clinic that will give you medical care, even if you have no medical insurance or money.

Medline Plus
Website: http://www.nlm.nih.gov/medlineplus/directories.html
Find health professionals and facilities.

Revolution Health
P.O. Box 1615
Oldsmar, FL 34677-1615
Email: customercare@revolutionhealth.com
Website: http://www.revolutionhealth.com/care-providers

Locate health professionals and facilities.

Veterans Health Administration
Website: http://www1.va.gov/directory/guide/home.asp
Education (GI Bill): (888) 442-4551
VA Benefits: (800) 827-1000
Health Care Benefits: (877) 222-8387
Income Verification and Means Testing: (800) 929-8387
Life Insurance: (800) 669-8477
Mammography Helpline: (888) 492-7844
Special Issues—Gulf War/Agent Orange/Project Shad/Mustard
Agents and Lewisite/Ionizing Radiation: (800) 749-8387

The mission of the Veterans Healthcare System is to serve the
needs of America's veterans by providing primary care, specialized
care, and related medical and social support services.

Social Service Agencies and Other Nonprofit Resources

American Association of Retired Persons (AARP)
Telephone Number: (202) 434-2277 or (888) 687-2277
Website: http://www.aarp.org/

This nonprofit membership organization is a good source of information on long-term care options, caregiving, legal and financial
planning, Medicare and Medicaid, and legislative issues affecting
the elderly.

ARCH National Respite Network
800 Eastowne Drive, Suite 105
Chapel Hill, NC 27514
Website: http://chtop.org/ARCH.html

Provides information on temporary relief for caregivers and families who are caring for those with disabilities, chronic or terminal illnesses, or the elderly.

Catholic Charities USA
Sixty-Six Canal Center Plaza, Suite 600
Alexandria, VA 22314
Telephone Number: (703) 549-1390
Fax Number: (703) 549-1656
Website: http://www.catholiccharitiesusa.org/

Catholic Charities agencies and institutions nationwide provide vital social services to people in need, regardless of their religious, social or economic backgrounds.

Jewish Board of Family and Children's Services
120 West 57th Street
New York, NY 10019
Telephone Number: (212) 582-9100 or (888) 523-2769
http://www.jbfcs.org/
Website: http://www.jbfcs.org/

One of the nation's largest and most respected nonprofit mental health and social service agencies serving over 65,000 New Yorkers annually from all religious, ethnic and economic backgrounds through 185 community-based programs, residential facilities and day-treatment centers.

National Alliance for Hispanic Health
1501 Sixteenth Street, N.W.
Washington, DC 20036
Telephone Number: (202) 387-5000
Website: http://www.hispanichealth.org/

The National Alliance for Hispanic Health is the premier organization focusing on Hispanic health. Alliance members reach over 14 million Hispanic consumers throughout the United States.

Volunteers of America
1660 Duke Street
Alexandria, VA 22314
Telephone Number: (703) 341-5000
Fax Number: (703) 341-7000
Website: http://www.voa.org/

Volunteers of America is a major provider of professional long-term nursing care for seniors and others coping with illness or injury. They offer a continuum of services that includes assisted living, memory care, nursing care, rehabilitative therapy and more.

Online Support Groups or Web Forums

CareCentral
1655 N. Fort Myer Drive, Suite 400
Arlington, VA 22209
Telephone Number: (703) 302-1040
Fax Number: (703) 248-0830
Website: http://www.carecentral.com/

CareCentral allows you or your loved one to create your own personalized website to provide friends and families with a central hub to keep in touch, stay informed, and share support during important events in your life.

CaringBridge

1995 Rahn Cliff Court, Suite 200
Eagan, MN 55122
Telephone Number: (651) 452-7940
Website: http://www.caringbridge.org/

CaringBridge is a nonprofit organization offering free personalized websites to those wishing to stay in touch with family and friends during significant life events.

Lotsa Helping Hands

365 Boston Post Road, Suite 157
Sudbury, MA 01776
Email: information@lotsahelpinghands.com
Website: http:// www.lotsahelpinghands.com

Provides online an easy-to-use, private group calendar, specifically designed for organizing helpers, where everyone can pitch in with meals delivery, rides, and other tasks necessary for life to run smoothly during a crisis.

Send Us Your Story

Do you have a story to tell? LaChance Publishing and The Healing Project publish four books a year of stories written by people like you. Have you or those you know been touched by life-threatening illness or chronic disease? Your story can give comfort, courage and strength to others who are going through what you have already faced.

Your story should be no less than 500 words and no more than 2,000 words. You can write about yourself or someone you know. Your story must inform, inspire or teach others. Tell the story of how you or someone you know faced adversity; what you learned that would be important for others to know; how dealing with the disease strengthened or clarified your relationships or inspired positive changes in your life.

The easiest way to submit your story is to visit the LaChance Publishing website at www.lachancepublishing.com. There you will find guidelines for submitting your story online, or you may write to us at submissions@lachancepublishing.com. We look forward to reading your story!